Polycystic Ovarian Syndrome

A Medical Dictionary, Bibliography,
and Annotated Research Guide to
Internet References

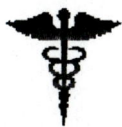

James N. Parker, M.D.
and Philip M. Parker, Ph.D., Editors

ICON Health Publications
ICON Group International, Inc.
4370 La Jolla Village Drive, 4th Floor
San Diego, CA 92122 USA

Copyright ©2004 by ICON Group International, Inc.

Copyright ©2004 by ICON Group International, Inc. All rights reserved. This book is protected by copyright. No part of it may be reproduced, stored in a retrieval system, or transmitted in any form or by any means, electronic, mechanical, photocopying, recording, or otherwise, without written permission from the publisher.

Printed in the United States of America.

Last digit indicates print number: 10 9 8 7 6 4 5 3 2 1

Publisher, Health Care: Philip Parker, Ph.D.
Editor(s): James Parker, M.D., Philip Parker, Ph.D.

Publisher's note: The ideas, procedures, and suggestions contained in this book are not intended for the diagnosis or treatment of a health problem. As new medical or scientific information becomes available from academic and clinical research, recommended treatments and drug therapies may undergo changes. The authors, editors, and publisher have attempted to make the information in this book up to date and accurate in accord with accepted standards at the time of publication. The authors, editors, and publisher are not responsible for errors or omissions or for consequences from application of the book, and make no warranty, expressed or implied, in regard to the contents of this book. Any practice described in this book should be applied by the reader in accordance with professional standards of care used in regard to the unique circumstances that may apply in each situation. The reader is advised to always check product information (package inserts) for changes and new information regarding dosage and contraindications before prescribing any drug or pharmacological product. Caution is especially urged when using new or infrequently ordered drugs, herbal remedies, vitamins and supplements, alternative therapies, complementary therapies and medicines, and integrative medical treatments.

Cataloging-in-Publication Data

Parker, James N., 1961-
Parker, Philip M., 1960-

Polycystic Ovarian Syndrome: A Medical Dictionary, Bibliography, and Annotated Research Guide to Internet References / James N. Parker and Philip M. Parker, editors
        p.   cm.
Includes bibliographical references, glossary, and index.
ISBN: 0-597-84171-3
1. Polycystic Ovarian Syndrome-Popular works.   I. Title.

Disclaimer

This publication is not intended to be used for the diagnosis or treatment of a health problem. It is sold with the understanding that the publisher, editors, and authors are not engaging in the rendering of medical, psychological, financial, legal, or other professional services.

References to any entity, product, service, or source of information that may be contained in this publication should not be considered an endorsement, either direct or implied, by the publisher, editors, or authors. ICON Group International, Inc., the editors, and the authors are not responsible for the content of any Web pages or publications referenced in this publication.

Copyright Notice

If a physician wishes to copy limited passages from this book for patient use, this right is automatically granted without written permission from ICON Group International, Inc. (ICON Group). However, all of ICON Group publications have copyrights. With exception to the above, copying our publications in whole or in part, for whatever reason, is a violation of copyright laws and can lead to penalties and fines. Should you want to copy tables, graphs, or other materials, please contact us to request permission (E-mail: iconedit@san.rr.com). ICON Group often grants permission for very limited reproduction of our publications for internal use, press releases, and academic research. Such reproduction requires confirmed permission from ICON Group International, Inc. **The disclaimer above must accompany all reproductions, in whole or in part, of this book.**

Acknowledgements

The collective knowledge generated from academic and applied research summarized in various references has been critical in the creation of this book which is best viewed as a comprehensive compilation and collection of information prepared by various official agencies which produce publications on polycystic ovarian syndrome. Books in this series draw from various agencies and institutions associated with the United States Department of Health and Human Services, and in particular, the Office of the Secretary of Health and Human Services (OS), the Administration for Children and Families (ACF), the Administration on Aging (AOA), the Agency for Healthcare Research and Quality (AHRQ), the Agency for Toxic Substances and Disease Registry (ATSDR), the Centers for Disease Control and Prevention (CDC), the Food and Drug Administration (FDA), the Healthcare Financing Administration (HCFA), the Health Resources and Services Administration (HRSA), the Indian Health Service (IHS), the institutions of the National Institutes of Health (NIH), the Program Support Center (PSC), and the Substance Abuse and Mental Health Services Administration (SAMHSA). In addition to these sources, information gathered from the National Library of Medicine, the United States Patent Office, the European Union, and their related organizations has been invaluable in the creation of this book. Some of the work represented was financially supported by the Research and Development Committee at INSEAD. This support is gratefully acknowledged. Finally, special thanks are owed to Tiffany Freeman for her excellent editorial support.

About the Editors

James N. Parker, M.D.

Dr. James N. Parker received his Bachelor of Science degree in Psychobiology from the University of California, Riverside and his M.D. from the University of California, San Diego. In addition to authoring numerous research publications, he has lectured at various academic institutions. Dr. Parker is the medical editor for health books by ICON Health Publications.

Philip M. Parker, Ph.D.

Philip M. Parker is the Eli Lilly Chair Professor of Innovation, Business and Society at INSEAD (Fontainebleau, France and Singapore). Dr. Parker has also been Professor at the University of California, San Diego and has taught courses at Harvard University, the Hong Kong University of Science and Technology, the Massachusetts Institute of Technology, Stanford University, and UCLA. Dr. Parker is the associate editor for ICON Health Publications.

About ICON Health Publications

To discover more about ICON Health Publications, simply check with your preferred online booksellers, including Barnes&Noble.com and Amazon.com which currently carry all of our titles. Or, feel free to contact us directly for bulk purchases or institutional discounts:

>ICON Group International, Inc.
>4370 La Jolla Village Drive, Fourth Floor
>San Diego, CA 92122 USA
>Fax: 858-546-4341
>Web site: **www.icongrouponline.com/health**

Table of Contents

FORWARD	1
CHAPTER 1. STUDIES ON POLYCYSTIC OVARIAN SYNDROME	3
Overview	*3*
The Combined Health Information Database	*3*
Federally Funded Research on Polycystic Ovarian Syndrome	*5*
E-Journals: PubMed Central	*26*
The National Library of Medicine: PubMed	*27*
CHAPTER 2. NUTRITION AND POLYCYSTIC OVARIAN SYNDROME	69
Overview	*69*
Finding Nutrition Studies on Polycystic Ovarian Syndrome	*69*
Federal Resources on Nutrition	*76*
Additional Web Resources	*77*
CHAPTER 3. ALTERNATIVE MEDICINE AND POLYCYSTIC OVARIAN SYNDROME	79
Overview	*79*
National Center for Complementary and Alternative Medicine	*79*
Additional Web Resources	*83*
General References	*84*
CHAPTER 4. DISSERTATIONS ON POLYCYSTIC OVARIAN SYNDROME	85
Overview	*85*
Dissertations on Polycystic Ovarian Syndrome	*85*
Keeping Current	*86*
CHAPTER 5. CLINICAL TRIALS AND POLYCYSTIC OVARIAN SYNDROME	87
Overview	*87*
Recent Trials on Polycystic Ovarian Syndrome	*87*
Keeping Current on Clinical Trials	*89*
CHAPTER 6. PATENTS ON POLYCYSTIC OVARIAN SYNDROME	91
Overview	*91*
Patents on Polycystic Ovarian Syndrome	*91*
Patent Applications on Polycystic Ovarian Syndrome	*94*
Keeping Current	*97*
CHAPTER 7. BOOKS ON POLYCYSTIC OVARIAN SYNDROME	99
Overview	*99*
Book Summaries: Online Booksellers	*99*
The National Library of Medicine Book Index	*100*
Chapters on Polycystic Ovarian Syndrome	*100*
CHAPTER 8. MULTIMEDIA ON POLYCYSTIC OVARIAN SYNDROME	103
Overview	*103*
Bibliography: Multimedia on Polycystic Ovarian Syndrome	*103*
CHAPTER 9. PERIODICALS AND NEWS ON POLYCYSTIC OVARIAN SYNDROME	105
Overview	*105*
News Services and Press Releases	*105*
Academic Periodicals covering Polycystic Ovarian Syndrome	*107*
APPENDIX A. PHYSICIAN RESOURCES	111
Overview	*111*
NIH Guidelines	*111*
NIH Databases	*113*
Other Commercial Databases	*115*
The Genome Project and Polycystic Ovarian Syndrome	*115*
APPENDIX B. PATIENT RESOURCES	119
Overview	*119*
Patient Guideline Sources	*119*

Finding Associations *123*
APPENDIX C. FINDING MEDICAL LIBRARIES 125
Overview *125*
Preparation *125*
Finding a Local Medical Library *125*
Medical Libraries in the U.S. and Canada *125*

ONLINE GLOSSARIES 131

Online Dictionary Directories *132*

POLYCYSTIC OVARIAN SYNDROME DICTIONARY 135

INDEX 185

FORWARD

In March 2001, the National Institutes of Health issued the following warning: "The number of Web sites offering health-related resources grows every day. Many sites provide valuable information, while others may have information that is unreliable or misleading."[1] Furthermore, because of the rapid increase in Internet-based information, many hours can be wasted searching, selecting, and printing. Since only the smallest fraction of information dealing with polycystic ovarian syndrome is indexed in search engines, such as **www.google.com** or others, a non-systematic approach to Internet research can be not only time consuming, but also incomplete. This book was created for medical professionals, students, and members of the general public who want to know as much as possible about polycystic ovarian syndrome, using the most advanced research tools available and spending the least amount of time doing so.

In addition to offering a structured and comprehensive bibliography, the pages that follow will tell you where and how to find reliable information covering virtually all topics related to polycystic ovarian syndrome, from the essentials to the most advanced areas of research. Public, academic, government, and peer-reviewed research studies are emphasized. Various abstracts are reproduced to give you some of the latest official information available to date on polycystic ovarian syndrome. Abundant guidance is given on how to obtain free-of-charge primary research results via the Internet. **While this book focuses on the field of medicine, when some sources provide access to non-medical information relating to polycystic ovarian syndrome, these are noted in the text.**

E-book and electronic versions of this book are fully interactive with each of the Internet sites mentioned (clicking on a hyperlink automatically opens your browser to the site indicated). If you are using the hard copy version of this book, you can access a cited Web site by typing the provided Web address directly into your Internet browser. You may find it useful to refer to synonyms or related terms when accessing these Internet databases. **NOTE:** At the time of publication, the Web addresses were functional. However, some links may fail due to URL address changes, which is a common occurrence on the Internet.

For readers unfamiliar with the Internet, detailed instructions are offered on how to access electronic resources. For readers unfamiliar with medical terminology, a comprehensive glossary is provided. For readers without access to Internet resources, a directory of medical libraries, that have or can locate references cited here, is given. We hope these resources will prove useful to the widest possible audience seeking information on polycystic ovarian syndrome.

The Editors

---

[1] From the NIH, National Cancer Institute (NCI): http://www.cancer.gov/cancerinfo/ten-things-to-know.

CHAPTER 1. STUDIES ON POLYCYSTIC OVARIAN SYNDROME

Overview

In this chapter, we will show you how to locate peer-reviewed references and studies on polycystic ovarian syndrome.

The Combined Health Information Database

The Combined Health Information Database summarizes studies across numerous federal agencies. To limit your investigation to research studies and polycystic ovarian syndrome, you will need to use the advanced search options. First, go to **http://chid.nih.gov/index.html**. From there, select the "Detailed Search" option (or go directly to that page with the following hyperlink: **http://chid.nih.gov/detail/detail.html**). The trick in extracting studies is found in the drop boxes at the bottom of the search page where "You may refine your search by." Select the dates and language you prefer, and the format option "Journal Article." At the top of the search form, select the number of records you would like to see (we recommend 100) and check the box to display "whole records." We recommend that you type "polycystic ovarian syndrome" (or synonyms) into the "For these words:" box. Consider using the option "anywhere in record" to make your search as broad as possible. If you want to limit the search to only a particular field, such as the title of the journal, then select this option in the "Search in these fields" drop box. The following is what you can expect from this type of search:

- **Obesity: Is There Effective Treatment Now?**

    Source: Consultant. 37(11): 2945-2948, 2950-2953, 2957. November 1997.

    Contact: Available from Cliggott Publishing Company. 55 Holly Hill Lane, Box 4010, Greenwich, CT 06831-0010.

    Summary: This article begins by presenting data on the prevalence of obesity and identifying the risks and costs associated with it. This is followed by a discussion of the genetic, endocrine, metabolic, psychological, and environmental factors that may contribute to obesity. The article then describes the workup of obese patients and highlights findings that may indicate comorbid conditions or endocrine abnormalities such as hypothyroidism, Cushing's syndrome, **polycystic ovarian syndrome,** and insulin resistance. The evaluation of obesity involves a careful history taking and physical examination. In some patients, indirect calorimetry may be helpful for measuring resting energy expenditure and estimating calorie needs for weight loss. Using a nutritional supplement to achieve a defined caloric intake for a brief period can help patients by showing them that they can lose weight without resorting to caloric restriction below their resting energy expenditure. In addition, the article presents a weight management program based on lifestyle changes, including regular exercise and increased intake of whole grains, fruits, and vegetables. This program, known as Eat Right, incorporates a low fat, high fiber diet, exercise, and behavior modification. The program is suitable for most patients, including those who have diabetes. 6 tables. 33 references. (AA-M).

- **Type 2 Diabetes in Children and Adolescents**

Source: Diabetes Care. 23(3): 381-389. March 2000.

Contact: Available from American Diabetes Association. 1701 North Beauregard Street, Alexandria, VA 22311. (800) 232-3472. Website: www.diabetes.org.

Summary: This article presents the consensus position on type 2 diabetes in children and adolescents that resulted from a consensus development conference convened by the American Diabetes Association (ADA) in 1999. The consensus position deals with the issues of the epidemiology, classification, pathophysiology, treatment, and prevention of diabetes in children and adolescents and identifies the population of children and adolescents who should be tested for diabetes. The national prevalence for all types of diabetes is estimated to be 4.1 per 1,000 in Americans 12 to 19 years old. Evidence suggests that type 2 diabetes is increasing in children and adolescents. The initial classification of diabetes in children and adolescents is usually based on the clinical features at presentation. Children who have type 1 diabetes are not usually overweight and have recent weight loss, polyuria, and polydipsia. In contrast, most children who have type 2 diabetes are overweight or obese at diagnosis and present with glycosuria without ketonuria, absent or mild polyuria and polydipsia, and little or no weight loss. Other clinical features that suggest type 2 diabetes include a family history of diabetes and the presence of acanthosis nigricans and **polycystic ovarian syndrome.** Maturity onset diabetes of the young is a rare form of diabetes in children with a broad clinical spectrum that ranges from asymptomatic hyperglycemia to a severe acute presentation. Type 2 diabetes is a complex metabolic disorder of heterogeneous etiology with social, behavioral, and environmental risk factors. There is a strong hereditary component to the disease, and puberty appears to play a major role in its development in children. The ADA recommends that only children at substantial risk for the presence or the development of type 2 diabetes should be tested. Risk factors that indicate the need for testing include being overweight, having a family history of type 2 diabetes, belonging to a certain race or ethnic group, and having signs of insulin resistance or conditions associated with insulin resistance. Suitable tests for diagnosing diabetes are the fasting plasma glucose test and the 2 hour plasma glucose test. Treatment involves providing all children who have type 2 diabetes with comprehensive self management education. Other therapeutic components include self monitoring blood glucose, modifying eating habits, and increasing daily physical activity. Pharmaceutical therapy with glucose lowering oral agents or insulin may also be needed. Types of oral agents currently available in the United States for the treatment of type 2 diabetes include biguanides, sulfonylureas, meglitinide, glucosidase inhibitors, and thiazolidenediones. Lifestyle modifications focusing on weight management and increasing physical activity made at an early stage in high risk individuals might delay or prevent the onset of type 2 diabetes. 1 figure. 4 tables. 20 references.

- **Type 2 Diabetes in Children and Adolescents: An Emerging Disease**

    Source: Journal of Pediatric Health Care. 15(4): 187-193. July-August 2001.

    Contact: Available from Mosby. 6277 Sea Harbor Drive, Orlando, FL 32887. (800) 654-2452 or (407) 345-4000. Fax (407) 363-9661.

    Summary: This review article presents pediatric nurse practitioners with the most recent information about type 2 diabetes in children and adolescents, summarizes current understanding about diagnosis, and outlines treatment options. Although children and adolescents are usually diagnosed with type 1 diabetes, within the past 10 years children as young as 8 years old have been diagnosed with the type 2 diabetes. Type 2 diabetes in youth is an emerging disease, so its natural history is not well understood. Risk factors for type 2 diabetes in children and adolescents are similar to those in adults, including non-European ancestry, family history of type 2 diabetes, obesity, insulin resistance, and age. African American and Hispanic youth are at greater risk than white youth. The initial assessment of children and adolescents with a potential diagnosis of diabetes is critical. Although youth with type 2 diabetes may or may not have the classic symptoms of polydipsia, polyuria, and polyphagia, they often have features associated with insulin resistance syndrome such as dyslipidemia, hyperglycemia, obesity, hypertension, **polycystic ovarian syndrome,** and acanthosis nigricans. Blood glucose levels are essential to the diagnosis of diabetes, but additional laboratory measures are also important. The aim of treatment is to normalize blood glucose and glycosylated hemoglobin values. Fundamental to this aim is an individualized plan for nutrition and activity. The choice of pharmacologic management will depend on the child's clinical presentation. Currently, insulin and metformin are the only drugs approved by the Food and Drug Administration for the treatment of diabetes in children; however, selected oral medications have been used with success. Diabetes self management education is also an essential component in the management of diabetes. Education must focus on psychomotor skills, medical nutrition therapy, and physical activity. Routine follow up care should occur every 3 to 4 months. Primary prevention activities include counseling all patients about the importance of a healthy diet and exercise and monitoring physical development. The article presents a case study and discusses the nursing and research implications of type 2 diabetes in youth. 1 figure. 2 tables. 28 references. (AA-M).

Federally Funded Research on Polycystic Ovarian Syndrome

The U.S. Government supports a variety of research studies relating to polycystic ovarian syndrome. These studies are tracked by the Office of Extramural Research at the National Institutes of Health.[2] CRISP (Computerized Retrieval of Information on Scientific Projects) is a searchable database of federally funded biomedical research projects conducted at universities, hospitals, and other institutions.

---

[2] Healthcare projects are funded by the National Institutes of Health (NIH), Substance Abuse and Mental Health Services (SAMHSA), Health Resources and Services Administration (HRSA), Food and Drug Administration (FDA), Centers for Disease Control and Prevention (CDCP), Agency for Healthcare Research and Quality (AHRQ), and Office of Assistant Secretary of Health (OASH).

Search the CRISP Web site at **http://crisp.cit.nih.gov/crisp/crisp_query.generate_screen**. You will have the option to perform targeted searches by various criteria, including geography, date, and topics related to polycystic ovarian syndrome.

For most of the studies, the agencies reporting into CRISP provide summaries or abstracts. As opposed to clinical trial research using patients, many federally funded studies use animals or simulated models to explore polycystic ovarian syndrome. The following is typical of the type of information found when searching the CRISP database for polycystic ovarian syndrome:

- **Project Title: ADRENAL ANDROGEN EXCESS IN THE POLYCYSTIC OVARY SYNDROME**

    Principal Investigator & Institution: Azziz, Ricardo; Professor and Chairman; Obstetrics and Gynecology; University of Alabama at Birmingham Uab Station Birmingham, Al 35294

    Timing: Fiscal Year 2001; Project Start 01-MAY-1993; Project End 30-NOV-2002

    Summary: Adrenal androgen (AA) production is frequently abnormal in women with hyperandrogenic oligoovulation (HO). A number of investigators, including ourselves, have noted that AA excess may result from a generalized adrenocortical hyper-reactivity to adrenocorticotropic hormone (ACTH) or pituitary overresponse to corticotropin releasing hormone (CRH). This adrenocortical dysfunction may represent an acquired defect secondary to excessive ovarian secretion of androgens, such as testosterone. Alternatively, the dysfunction may represent an inherited abnormality, such as heterozygosity for 21-hydroxylase (21-OH) deficiency. Regardless of the etiology, the significance of AA excess in the maintenance of ovulatory dysfunction in HO is unclear. The Specific Aims of the proposal include: 1) to establish the sensitivity and responsivity to ACTH and CRH in HO patients with and without adrenocortical dysfunction; 2) to establish the role of ovarian factors in the development/maintenance of adrenocortical dysfunction; 3) to establish the role of mild inherited defects in adrenal 21-OH function in the development of HO; 4) and to establish the role of AA excess in the maintenance of ovulatory dysfunction in HO patients, while elucidating endocrine markers for a favorable response to corticosteroid suppression. To achieve Specific Aim 1 the adrenocortical sensitivity and responsivity to incremental doses of ACTH, and to ovine CRH, will be determined in 10 HO patients with and 10 without adrenocortical hyperreactivity, and in 10 control women. For Specific Aim 2 ten HO patients with and 10 without adrenocortical dysfunction will undergo three months of ovarian suppression using a long-acting GnRH-a, and alterations in basal androgen profiles, response to ovine CRH and ACTH, and glucose tolerance will be assessed. For Specific Aim 3 at least 30 females who are obligate heterozygotes for 21-OH deficiency will be studied for the presence of HO. To achieve Specific Aim 4 at least forty consecutive patients presenting with HO will be treated with three months of dexamethasone (0.5 mg/day), and their clinical response correlated with various adrenocortical markers. These studies will shed light on the etiology and role of adrenocortical of HO.

    Website: http://crisp.cit.nih.gov/crisp/Crisp_Query.Generate_Screen

- **Project Title: ANDROGENS AND SUBCLINICAL ATHEROSCLEROSIS IN YOUNG WOMEN**

    Principal Investigator & Institution: Siscovick, David S.; Medicine; University of Washington Seattle, Wa 98195

    Timing: Fiscal Year 2001; Project Start 30-SEP-2001; Project End 31-JUL-2004

Summary: (provided by applicant): This revised application represents an ancillary study to the Coronary Artery Risk Development in Young Adults (CARDIA) Study, a large cohort study supported by the NHLBI. Several studies have demonstrated cross-sectional associations of hyperandrogenism, the primary biochemical feature of clinically-diagnosed **polycystic ovarian syndrome** (PCOS), with coronary risk factors and atherosclerosis. We propose to examine whether serum androgens, measured earlier in life, and variation in genes related to androgen synthesis, metabolism, and signaling are associated with early-onset subclinical coronary atherosclerosis in young adult women from the community. Additionally, we will examine whether the clinical features of PCOS are associated with subclinical coronary atherosclerosis in young adult women, after taking into account serum androgens. CARDIA provides a unique platform to address these questions; and, the proposed ancillary study will add the laboratory and clinical measurements to CARDIA needed to examine these questions. In the prospective component of the proposed study, we will examine the associations of serum androgens and genetic polymorphisms and haplotypes in ten candidate genes with the presence of coronary artery calcium (CAC) by CT. Androgen and genotyping measures will be made using stored serum and DNA samples collected from 1550 women 5 and 13 years prior to the assessment of CAC at age 33 to 45 years. In the cross-sectional component, we will use information collected at a proposed ancillary study visit in Year 16 to examine the associations of the clinical features of PCOS, including the presence of **polycystic ovaries** detected using trans-vaginal ultrasound, menstrual irregularities, infertility, and hirsutism, with the presence of CAC at Year 15 (n= 1200). Secondarily, we will determine whether longitudinal changes in obesity, physical inactivity, and insulin levels influence the prospective associations of serum androgens and genetic variants in candidate genes with subclinical coronary atherosclerosis. In short, the proposed study addresses a potentially important and relatively unexplored area of investigation related to women's cardiovascular health.

Website: http://crisp.cit.nih.gov/crisp/Crisp_Query.Generate_Screen

- **Project Title: CLINICAL & BASIC STUDIES IN POLYCYSTIC OVARIAN SYNDROME**

    Principal Investigator & Institution: Marshall, John C.; Arthur and Margaret Ebbert; Internal Medicine; University of Virginia Charlottesville Box 400195 Charlottesville, Va 22904

    Timing: Fiscal Year 2001; Project Start 01-APR-1993; Project End 31-MAR-2003

    Summary: (Adapted from applicant's application) The proposed U54 Center at Virginia will have a major goal of promoting translational research leading to application of new basic findings to clinical application. The Center theme is "Clinical and Basic Studies in **Polycystic Ovarian Syndrome** (PCOS)." This topic is appropriate to the goals of the Cooperative Centers Program, in that present therapeutic approaches to the anovulation and metabolic abnormalities in the disorder are of limited efficacy, and importantly, the basic mechanisms underlying PCOS remain uncertain. Current hypothesis as to the etiology of PCOS center around regulation of GnRH secretion and action, and/or disordered ovarian function, either primary in nature or consequent to abnormal stimulation by gonadotropins or co-gonadotropins such as insulin and IGF-1. The U54 Center proposes 2 clinical and 2 related basic projects to investigate these areas. Project I addressed potential abnormalities in regulation of the GnRH pulse generator and is directly related to Project II, on cellular mechanisms of GnRH frequency regulation of gonadotropin gene expression. Project IV (contract with Virginia Commonwealth University), addresses the clinical effects of reduction of hyperinsulinemia on metabolic profiles and ovulation. Project V is directly related, addressing the mechanism of IGF-1 and LH synergism on ovarian theca cells. The Center subprojects are supported by 4 cores proposed to operated under an "open access" formula. Overall integration of the research will be performed by the Administration Core, and specific laboratory services will be available to U54 projects and to eligible funded RSB program relevant projects through molecular biology, cell science and ligand assay and analysis cores.

Website: http://crisp.cit.nih.gov/crisp/Crisp_Query.Generate_Screen

- **Project Title: COOPERATIVE MULTI CENTER REPRODUCTIVE MEDICINE NETWORK**

    Principal Investigator & Institution: Myers, Evan R.; Associate Professor; Obstetrics and Gynecology; Duke University Durham, Nc 27706

    Timing: Fiscal Year 2001; Project Start 10-MAR-2000; Project End 28-FEB-2005

    Summary: Disorders of the reproductive system, such as male and female infertility, leiomyomata, endometriosis, **polycystic ovarian syndrome,** and sexual dysfunction, have a major public health and economic impact. For some conditions, such as infertility, many patients are responsible for all costs associated with therapy, and unintended consequences, such as multiple gestations, are relatively common. For other conditions, such as endometriosis or leiomyomata, definitive therapy may result in the loss of childbearing potential, and long-term evidence about alternatives is scant. Relatively few interventions for these disorders have subjected to rigorous scientific evaluation. The long-term objective of this project is to improve the care of men and women with disorders affecting the reproductive system by conducting controlled trials of selected diagnostic and therapeutic interventions. The specific aims of the Data Coordinating Center (DCC) for the Cooperative Reproductive Medicine Network are (A) to develop trial protocols that address important clinical problems using scientifically valid, clinically feasible, and economically reasonable approaches through collaboration with participating Reproductive Medicine Units (RMUs) and NICHD staff, (B) to provide leadership in defining and measuring a range of important outcomes, including physiological measurements, clinical outcomes, and economic and quality of life measures, (C) to coordinate and/or provide all services necessary for conducting trials, including recruiting services, and quality control, and (D) to coordinate the analysis, reporting, and dissemination of trial results to the Data Safety and Monitoring Committee, the RMUs, NICHD, peer-reviewed journals, and the public.

    Website: http://crisp.cit.nih.gov/crisp/Crisp_Query.Generate_Screen

- **Project Title: EFFECTS OF DECREASED HYPERINSULINEMIA ON THE OVULATORY RESPONSE TO CLOMIPHENE**

    Principal Investigator & Institution: Vandermolen, David T.; Virginia Commonwealth University Richmond, Va 232980568

    Timing: Fiscal Year 2001

    Summary: To determine if patients with chronic anovulation due to **polycystic ovarian syndrome** who are clomiphene resistant will have an improved ovulatory response to clomiphene with correction of hyperinsulinemia.

    Website: http://crisp.cit.nih.gov/crisp/Crisp_Query.Generate_Screen

- **Project Title: ENDOMETRIAL INTEGRINS AND UTERINE RECEPTIVITY**

    Principal Investigator & Institution: Lessey, Bruce A.; University of North Carolina Chapel Hill Office of Sponsored Research Chapel Hill, Nc 27599

Timing: Fiscal Year 2002; Project Start 02-MAY-2002; Project End 31-MAR-2007

Summary: The study of implantation in the human has yielded convincing evidence for a defined period of uterine receptivity that is characterized by developmental changes on the surface epithelium of the endometrium. Using the integrin alpha-v beta-3 and its ligand osteopontin (OPN), we have described a pattern of expression for each that corresponds well with the time of implantation. We have studied he regulation of these proteins and found that each protein is independently regulated by two separate pathways, yet both pathways involve he coordinated action of estrogen and progesterone. **Polycystic ovarian syndrome** (PCOS) is a common endocrine problem in reproductive-aged women, resulting in infertility and frequent miscarriage. Our studies suggest that androgen receptors (ARs) and two p160 coactivators, AIB-1 and TIF2, are over- expressed in the endometrium of women with PCOS. These changes are associated with aberrant patterns of integrin expression and retarded endometrial development in ovulatory patients with this disorder. We hypothesize that the elevated AR and co-activator expression sensitizes the endometrium to weaker androgens and promotes androgen action in response to lower concentrations of strong androgens. Furthermore, other steroid hormones, such as estrogen or progesterone may activate AR or ER in response to elevated coactivator expression in these women. If this occurs, estrogen, which is a potent inhibitor of uterine receptivity, could interfere with the expression of critical genes during the time of maximal uterine receptivity. To investigate this important biologic question we propose 3 Aims: 1) To investigate the expression of alpha-5 beta-3 and its ligand OPN in normal and PCOS endometrium and to use these biomarkers to study the pathways that may render the endometrium of PCOS women infertile. Methods will include characterization of ERalpha and ERbeta, PR-A and PR-B and AR throughout the menstrual cycle, assessment of steroid regulation of alpha-5 beta-3 and OPN using their respective promoters, and in vitro techniques to study paracrine mechanisms of steroid action in the endometrium. 2) Prospectively study the expression of three p160 co- activators in the endometrial epithelial and stromal cells throughout the menstrual cycle in normal and PCOS endometrium. Using in vivo models we will investigate the consequences of coactivator over expression in these cells. 3) Using DNA microarray analysis, we plan to further characterize the altered pattern of gene expression in women with PCOS compared to normal cycling women. Knowing what changes occur in the endometrium of androgenized endometrium we hope to begin to better understand the mechanism of dysfunction that occurs. Validation of these changes will provide new avenues for research into the effects of androgens on the endometrium. The complex relationships between steroid receptors and their ligands and co-activators provide a framework to investigate the mechanisms by which uterine receptivity is regulated and dysregulated in certain infertility states.

Website: http://crisp.cit.nih.gov/crisp/Crisp_Query.Generate_Screen

- **Project Title: FETAL ANDROGEN INDUCES OVARIAN, LH AND B-CELL DEFECTS**

Principal Investigator & Institution: Abbott, David H.; Northwestern University 633 Clark St Evanston, Il 60208

Timing: Fiscal Year 2002; Project Start 01-SEP-2002; Project End 31-AUG-2007

Summary: Polycystic ovarian syndrome (PCOS) affects approximately 5-10% of reproductive aged women and is characterized by hyperandrogenic anovulation, early-onset type II diabetes mellitus, obesity, atherosclerosis and endometrial cancer. Hyperinsulinemia plays a key role in the mechanism of hyperandrogenic anovulation.

The etiology of PCOS in women, however, is unknown. Prenatal androgen excess in female rhesus monkeys results in ovarian, endocrinological and metabolic features in adulthood that closely resemble those found in women with PCOS. In Project #3 of this SCOR application, we propose to employ a unique non-human primate model of PCOS to define a fetal origin for the syndrome. We propose that hyprandrogenism, the core functional disorder in women with PCOS, reprograms multiple fetal organ systems in females resulting in the phenotypic expression of the syndrome. Recent findings of prevalent PCOS in women exposed to in utero androgen excess strongly support this hypothesis. Our preliminary results suggest that early exposure to androgen excess during gestation produces ovarian hyperandrogenism, LH hypersecretion and impaired pancreatic insulin secretion in adult animals. This project will [1] demonstrated increased fetal and neonatal LH hypersecretion in female rhesus monkeys following prenatal androgenization on Dys 40-80 of gestation (LH defect), [2] establish ovarian hyperandrogenism in fetal and neonatal PA female rhesus monkeys [ovarian defect], [3] characterize the neonatal ovaries removed from PA female rhesus monkeys for morphological abnormalities and changed mRNA expression indicative of hyperandrogenic phenotype [ovarian defect], [4] determine whether in utero testosterone (T) excess during Days 40-80 of gestation induces impaired fetal and neonatal pancreatic insulin secretion in female rhesus monkeys [beta0cell defect], [5] assess impairments in fetal and neonatal physical development induced by prenatal androgen excess. The project will also provide a complementary and experimental study to that in PCOS pregnancies in [Project #1] and will produce hypothalamic and pancreatic tissue to determine whether prenatal androgen excess in female rhesus monkeys results in profound suppression of KATP channel subunit expression [Project #4].

Website: http://crisp.cit.nih.gov/crisp/Crisp_Query.Generate_Screen

- **Project Title: FUNCTIONAL OVARIAN HYPERANDROGENISM/MINORITY ADOLESCENTS**

    Principal Investigator & Institution: Rieder, Jessica; Montefiore Medical Center (Bronx, Ny) Bronx, Ny 104672490

    Timing: Fiscal Year 2001; Project Start 01-AUG-2001; Project End 31-JUL-2003

    Summary: (provided by applicant): Functional Ovarian Hyperandrogenism (FOH), also called **Polycystic Ovarian Syndrome** (PCOS) consists of a spectrum of dysfunction with varying degrees of ovulatory dysfunction, hyperandrogenemia, and clinically evident hyperandrogenism. The biochemical and clinical criteria for hyperandrogenemia and hyperandrogenism have not yet been determined for a large ethnic minority female adolescent population. The specific aims of the study are: 1) to determine the relationship between the clinical presentation and the biochemical determinants of FOH/PCOS in a clinical sample of predominantly Caribbean-Hispanic and African-American female adolescents; 2) to establish norms for the biochemical determinants of hyperandrogenemia in this population; 3) to determine the clinical correlates of hyperandrogenemia in adolescent girls; and 4) to determine if adolescent females with FOH/PCOS are more likely than normal, weight-matched adolescents to be Caribbean-Hispanic, to have a family history of diabetes, high blood pressure or cardiovascular disease, or to have significantly higher glucose to insulin ratios. The hypotheses are as follows: 1) the testosterone and androstenedione levels in subjects with menstrual cycle abnormalities and/or physical evidence of hyperandrogenism will be significantly greater than in those with normal menstrual cycles and no physical evidence for hyperandrogenism; 2) a combination of clinical and historical features may be used to develop a model that can predict serum androgen levels; and 3) subjects with FOH/PCOS will be more likely than normal subjects to be of Caribbean-Hispanic descent, to have evidence of risk factors for diabetes mellitus and cardiovascular disease, and to have significantly higher glucose to insulin ratios. 250 females aged 12 to 21 will be consecutively recruited from several clinical sites; girls with chronic illnesses or on hormonally active drugs will be excluded. Subjects will complete a questionnaire to elicit features of menstrual and family history and will undergo a physical examination to evaluate for clinical signs of hyperandrogenism. Serum levels of fasting free and total testosterone, androstenedione, luteinizing hormone, follicle stimulating hormone, insulin, 17-OH progesterone, and glucose will be measured. To determine the association of serum androgen levels with clinical features of FOH/PCOS, all subjects will be clinically stratified into three different categories and androgen levels will be compared among these groups, using ANOVA. Hyperandrogenism will be defined as two standard deviations above the mean testosterone and androstenedione levels in subjects with normal menstrual cycles and no physical evidence of hyperandrogenism (category I). A clinical prediction model for hyperandrogenemia will be developed using multiple linear regression analyses for androgen measures. A case-control study will be performed to determine differences between adolescent subjects with and without FOH/PCOS. Improved understanding of the boichemical and clinical features of FOH/PCOS in minority adolescents will facilitate the development of earlier treatment modalities and prevention of later serious health problems that result from the natural progression of this disorder.

Website: http://crisp.cit.nih.gov/crisp/Crisp_Query.Generate_Screen

- **Project Title: GLUCOSE MEATBOLISM IN THE HUMAN OVARY**

    Principal Investigator & Institution: Charron, Maureen J.; Professor of Biochemistry; Biochemistry; Yeshiva University 500 W 185Th St New York, Ny 10033

    Timing: Fiscal Year 2003; Project Start 20-JAN-2003; Project End 31-DEC-2004

    Summary: (provided by applicant): GLUT4 is the main insulin responsive glucose transporter in adipose and muscle which plays an important role in regulating glucose metabolism. While not sensitive to regulation by sex steroids, GLUT4 is commonly decreased in insulin resistant states. GLUTx1, also known as GLUT8, is a recently discovered glucose transporter that appears to be sex steroid regulated. It is expressed in human ovary and inhibited by sex steroids in human testis. These results suggest a sex steroid regulation of GLUT8 expression and a possible involvement of GLUT8 in the provision of glucose required for metabolic processes and DNA synthesis in germ cells. Glucose transport activity, could be an important determinant of metabolic as well as reproductive function in women. Alterations in peripheral as well as ovarian glucose transporters could be directly related to insulin resistance and perhaps to reproductive dysfunction. The relative expression of peripheral and ovarian GLUT4 and GLUT8 in women with **Polycystic Ovarian Syndrome** (PCOS) and normally cycling women has only partially been characterized. Alterations of GLUT8 and GLUT4 could provide insight into the pathophysiology of PCOS. To clarify the role of glucose transporters (e.g. GLUT8 and GLUT4) in normal and PCOS ovaries, the following Specific Aims are proposed. Aim 1 will examine the regulation of glucose transport and GLUT8 and GLUT4 expression/localization in a steroid-producing cell line to test the hypothesis that GLUT8, and not GLUT4, is sex steroid regulated within the ovary. Novel human ovarian theca-like and granulosa-like cell lines (HOTT and HGL-5 cells, respectively) will be used. Additionally, the ability of rosaglitazone (insulin sensitizer) to improve glucose uptake and transporter expression/localization in these cells will be assessed.

Aim 2 will determine the expression and cellular localization of glucose transporters in normal human ovary. Aim 3, concurrent with Aim 2, will test the hypothesis that the ovarian expression of GLUT8 and GLUT4 is decreased in women with PCOS relative to normally cycling age- and BMI-matched controls. Aims 2 and 3 will be carried out by a prospective, case-control study of women with PCOS undergoing ovarian drilling/wedge resection for fertility and a group of normally cycling women undergoing elective tubal sterilization. Immunohistochemistry, immunoblots and RT-PCR/real time PCR will be used to determine the expression and cellular localization of GLUT8 and GLUT4 in different tissues. The proposed studies are expected to provide mechanistic insight into the regulation of glucose transport within the ovary in women, an area that has been essentially unexplored. These observations are hoped to have relevance for understanding of basic reproductive physiology and the mechanism of reproductive dysfunction in PCOS.

Website: http://crisp.cit.nih.gov/crisp/Crisp_Query.Generate_Screen

- **Project Title: GLYCODELIN REGULATION IN POLYCYSTIC OVARIAN SYNDROME**

Principal Investigator & Institution: Taylor, Robert N.; Professor and Director; Ob, Gyn and Reproductive Scis; University of California San Francisco 500 Parnassus Ave San Francisco, Ca 94122

Timing: Fiscal Year 2003; Project Start 01-APR-2003; Project End 31-MAR-2007

Summary: (provided by applicant): Human embryonic implantation is a relatively unreliable process, failing in approximately 30% of conception cycles. One common condition associated with implantation failure is **polycystic ovary syndrome** (PCOS), which is the clinical focus of this application. Implantation is a complex and highly regulated process dependent upon precise endocrine and paracrine coordination of endometrial receptivity. Several proteins with diverse functions have been identified in the endometrial surface epithelium The expression of these proteins coincides with the timing of blastocyst attachment and trophoblast invasion. Ovarian hormones, and progesterone in particular, are believed to be the primary regulators of endometrial proteins expressed in the narrow window of implantation. Prior studies have established that glycodelin-A (GdA) is expressed in secretory phase and early pregnancy endometrial epithelium. GdA concentrations are decreased in cases with PCOS as well as in other causes of failed implantation and recurrent pregnancy loss. We discovered that GdA transcription is directly regulated by progestin-receptor complexes and that one of its biological activities is the inhibition of monocyte chemotaxis. Experiments proposed in this application are designed to evaluate the molecular mechanisms resulting in lower GdA production in PCOS. Laboratory experiments will establish the roles of androgens, luteinizing hormone (LH) and insulin on GdA biosynthesis in vitro models. GdA signaling and action in monocytes and other potential target cells will be evaluated. The GdA receptor will be purified and characterized. A case-control study of normal fertile women and women with PCOS will be conducted to dissect the potential pathways involved in GdA dysregulation in the latter group. Mock cycles will be induced and monitored by endometrial biopsies to determine the correlation of elevated androgens, LH and insulin to impaired GdA expression. Finally, a noninvasive quantitative evaluation of cervical fluid GdA will be developed as a potential marker for an "open" implantation window. Characterization of an optimal state for endometrial receptivity will have broad public health implications. Women suffering PCOS, infertility, recurrent pregnancy loss, and even later pregnancy complications such as preeclampsia and intrauterine growth restriction, will benefit from a better understanding of the cellular physiology of implantation and placentation.

Website: http://crisp.cit.nih.gov/crisp/Crisp_Query.Generate_Screen

- **Project Title: HYPOTHALAMIC-PITUITARY-OVARIAN AXIS IN WOMEN WITH EPILEPSY**

    Principal Investigator & Institution: Giudice, Linda C.; Stanford University Stanford, Ca 94305

    Timing: Fiscal Year 2001

    Summary: Women with epilepsy may be at risk for reproductive health dysfunctions, including menstrual irregularity, anovulation, **polycystic ovaries, polycystic ovarian syndrome,** and disturbances in basal and pulsatile release of gonadotropins and ovarian steroids. This study will define reproductive health risks for women with epilepsy and determine the relative mechanistic contribution of epilepsy syndrome, seizure frequency and type, and of individual antiepileptic drugs (AEDs) used in monotherapy. Pituitary and gonadal hormones, ovulatory function and ovarian morphology, and luteal phase function/adequacy will be evaluated in women with one of three distinct epilepsy syndromes: (1) idiopathic primary generalized epilepsy, in which the cerebral cortex is structurally and functionally normal: (2) symptomatic, localization related epilepsy (LRE) of temporal lobe origin, in which there is a structural and/or functional lesion within the temporal lobe; and (3) LRE of extratemporal lobe origin in which the epileptogenic region resides outside of the temporal lobe. These indices of reproductive function will also be evaluated according to exposure to AEDs in monotherapy that either induce, inhibit, or do not alter the hepatic mixed-function cytochrome P450 enzyme system. Women with LRE of temporal lobe origin are hypothesized to be preferentially at risk for reproductive health dysfunctions because, given the extensive input of the mesial temporal lobe to the hypothalamus, the temporal lobe epileptogenic lesion is likely to cause hypothalamic-pituitary axis dysfunction. Women with seizures involving the temporal lobe are also at risk since these seizures are associated with pituitary hormone abnormalities. In addition, AEDs which inhibit P450 will increase steroid hormone concentrations and may predispose to reproductive dysfunctions. The effects of temporal lobe epilepsy versus AEDs will be further differentiated by evaluating reproductive function in women before and after surgical resection of a temporal lobe epileptogenic focus, after which seizures are likely to remit while AEDs are held constant. These findings will permit the clinician to select an AED which is least likely to compromise reproductive health for a given epilepsy syndrome, and will make it more likely that women with epilepsy and reproductive dysfunction are identified and appropriately treated.

    Website: http://crisp.cit.nih.gov/crisp/Crisp_Query.Generate_Screen

- **Project Title: IGF-I SIGNALING IN GRANULOSA CELLS**

    Principal Investigator & Institution: Davis, John S.; Professor and Director of Research and d; Obstetrics and Gynecology; University of Nebraska Medical Center Omaha, Ne 681987835

    Timing: Fiscal Year 2001; Project Start 01-MAY-2001; Project End 31-JUL-2005

    Summary: (Scanned from the applicant's abstract) The intrafollicular IGF-I system amplifies gonadotropin hormone action in granulosa cells. IGF-I alone or in combination with FSH can induce gonadotropin receptors, steroidogenic enzymes and promote follicular survival. The important interplay among IGF-I and FSH is underscored by the striking similarity of ovaries in IGF-I knockout, FSH knockout and FSH receptor knockout mice. The follicles in these mice are arrested in the early antral stage of development. Whereas the mechanism of action of FSH is well known to involve the cAMP/protein kinase A signaling pathway, almost nothing is known about the intracellular actions of IGF-I in the ovary. Furthermore, recent studies by others and our preliminary data suggest that some of the signaling pathways utilized by IGF-I and FSH converge. The proposed studies are designed to test the overall hypothesis that IGF-I induced P1-3-kinase signaling pathway is required for granulosa cell survival and amplification of FSH-induced granulosa cell differentiation. The specific questions to be answered in this proposal are: Aim 1) Are the signaling events initiated by IGF-I amplified in response to FSH? Hypothesis: The IGF-I dependent P1-3-kinase signaling pathway in granulosa cells is augmented by FSH. Aim 2) Are the survival effects of IGF-I and FSH mediated by parallel or converging intracellular signaling pathways? Hypothesis I: The survival effects of IGF-I and FSH are mediated by P1-3-kinase/Akt mediated phosphorylation of Bad. Hypothesis II: IGF-I and FSH elevate the cellular ratio of antiapoptotic (e.g., Bc12, Bcl-Xlong, Mci-I) to pro-apoptotic proteins (e.g., Bad, Bax, Bok) and inhibit caspase activity. Aim 3) Is FSH directed granulosa cell differentiation mediated via IGF-I dependent signaling systems? Hypothesis: IGF-I stimulated P1-3-kinase signaling events amplifies FSH directed expression of differentiation, whereas ERK signaling represses djfferentiation. We will employ specific chemical inhibitors and adenovirus vectors that express dominant negative or active signaling molecules to dissect the IGF-I and FSH directed signaling pathways that are responsible for granulosa cell survival or granulosa cell differentiation. Further characterization of the IGF-I and FSH signaling events and their interactions are likely to provide new insights into how multiple genes are coordinately regulated by trophic factors during follicle development. Our studies are expected to translate into more effective treatments for controlling follicle selection and development, ovulation and fertility. This new insight may uncover mechanistic defects that underlay disorders of folliculogenesis, premature ovarian failure and disorders such as **polycystic ovarian syndrome.**

Website: http://crisp.cit.nih.gov/crisp/Crisp_Query.Generate_Screen

- **Project Title: INSULIN AND IGF-1 SIGNALING IN OVARIAN CELLS**

    Principal Investigator & Institution: Schomberg, David W.; Professor; Obstetrics and Gynecology; Duke University Durham, Nc 27706

    Timing: Fiscal Year 2001; Project Start 01-APR-2001; Project End 31-MAR-2003

    Summary: (Adapted from applicant's description): Our preliminary studies of ovaries from transgenic mice with a knockout of the insulin receptor substrate-1 gene (IRS-1 KO) showed entrapment of the oocyte in luteal tissue and that the number of animals ovulating was about one-third that of the wild-type (WT) control group. The IRS-1 KO ovaries also exhibited a rare phenotype, polyovular (bi-oocyte) follicles. These findings imply a relationship between compromised insulin signaling and phenotypic change in ovarian function which have not been previously recognized. Accordingly, the overall study objective is to validate and extend these findings to establish the role of insulin signaling pathway components at the ovarian level in vivo. With this background, detailed studies of how these effectors help execute the insulin- and Follicle-stimulating hormone-FSH) regulated end point alternatives of cell survival, apoptosis, or mitosis will proceed in an expanded application. The ovaries of WT and IRS-1 KO mice will be compared in various aspects in the following specific aims: 1) to evaluate oocyte numbers and biochemical markers in neonatal animals and the ovulatory response to exogenous gonadotropins in prepubertal animals, and 2) to assess levels and/or activity of early effectors in the insulin signaling pathway (IRS-1, IRS-2, P13-K, Akt) during gonadotropin-regulated follicular cell mitosis and apoptosis. Specific Aim 3 will extend the in vivo studies to in vitro analysis in cultured porcine granulosa cells (pGCs) to: a) examine possible connections between the FSH receptor and insulin/IGF-1 receptor signaling pathways, and b) develop improved methods to detect BAD (Bcl-2-associated death promoter), a critical regulator of cell fate which can be phosphorylated by Akt. The results obtained may also contribute information basic to a more complete understanding of an important clinical entity, **polycystic ovarian syndrome** (PCOS), which is characterized in part by accelerated follicle atresia (apoptosis), insulin resistance, and virilism.

Website: http://crisp.cit.nih.gov/crisp/Crisp_Query.Generate_Screen

- **Project Title: INSULIN AND THE POLYCYSTIC OVARY SYNDROME**

   Principal Investigator & Institution: Nestler, John E.; Professor and Chairman; Internal Medicine; Virginia Commonwealth University Richmond, Va 232980568

   Timing: Fiscal Year 2001; Project Start 01-AUG-1997; Project End 31-JUL-2005

   Summary: The polysystic ovary syndrome (PCOS) is a poorly understood disorder that affects approximately 6-10 percent of women of reproductive age. PCOS is characterized by hyperandrogenism and chronic anovulation, and is the leading cause of female infertility in the United States. Women with PCOS are also at high risk for developing type 2 diabetes, presumably due to the insulin resistance that accompanies the syndrome. Our long-term goal is to elucidate the relationship between insulin resistance and PCOS, especially as it relates to hyperandrogenism. Some actions of insulin may be effected by putative inositolphosphoglycan (IPG) mediators of insulin action and a deficiency in a specific D-chiro-inositol-containing IPG may contribute to insulin resistance in individuals with impaired glucose tolerance or type 2 diabetes. Our studies indicate that D-chiro-inositol (DCI) administration improves glucose intolerance while reducing circulating insulin in women with PCOS, and is also associated with decreases in serum androgens and improved ovulatory function. In addition, our in vitro studies in human thecal cell cultures suggest that the IPG signaling system plays a role in transducing insulin's stimulation of ovarian androgen biosynthesis. These studies have led us to focus our short- term goals on an assessment of the role of the IPG signaling system in PCOS, and pursue a unifying hypothesis to explain the above experimental observations. Our hypothesis is that women with PCOS are DCI deficient, perhaps related to an intracellular defect in the conversion of myo-inositol (MYO) to DCI. This results in a decrease in a DCI-containing IPG mediator (DCI-IPG) and an increase in a MYO-containing IPG mediator (MYO-IPG) bound to the outer leaflet of the cell membrane. We further propose that the resulting deficient insulin-mediated release of DCI-IPG contributes to insulin resistance in PCOS, whereas the simultaneous hyperinsulinemia mediated increased release of MYO-IPG at the level of the ovary acts to stimulate ovarian androgen biosynthesis. If our proposed studies confirm a role for IPG's in insulin resistance and hyperandrogenism of PCOS, they will substantially enhance our understanding of the disorder's pathogenesis and are likely to provide insights into novel treatment strategies directed specifically at the IPG system and normalization of its function.

   Website: http://crisp.cit.nih.gov/crisp/Crisp_Query.Generate_Screen

- **Project Title: INSULIN-INDUCED TRANSLOCATION OF GLUCOSE TRANSPORTER**

  Principal Investigator & Institution: Chi, Nai-Wen; Medicine; University of California San Diego 9500 Gilman Dr, Dept. 0934 La Jolla, Ca 92093

  Timing: Fiscal Year 2001; Project Start 30-SEP-1997; Project End 31-AUG-2003

  Summary: (Taken from the applicant's Abstract) Insulin plays an important role in glucose homeostasis by stimulating muscle and fat cells to take up glucose. Insulin does so by activating a signaling pathway that culminates in the recruitment of the glucose transporter GLUT4 from an intracellular compartment to the cell surface. This pathway apparently involves the activation of phosphatidylinositol 3-kinase (PI 3-kinase). However, the signaling target of PI 3-kinase remains unclear, and the effector machinery that translocates GLUT4 remains elusive. This insulin signaling pathway has significant medical implications, since its impairment may contribute to the development of obesity, diabetes mellitus, and **polycystic ovarian syndrome.** The long-term objective of the applicant is to understand in molecular terms how insulin works. Such knowledge may engender new treatments for the aforementioned diseases. The applicant proposes to address the following questions in cultured fat cells: 1. Does insulin-induced GLUT4 translocation involve the activation by PI 3-kinase of its proposed targets, such as protein kinase B and isoforms of protein kinase C? The role of these kineses will be investigated by activating or blocking them and observing the resultant effect on GLUT4 translocation. 2. Can insulin-induced GLUT4 translocation be explained by a putative intracellular GLUT4 chaperon? This chaperon would serve to anchor GLUT4 intracellularly in the absence of insulin. In the presence of insulin, the chaperon would release GLUT4 and allow it to follow the exocytic flow toward cell surface. To clone this putative chaperon, two strategies are proposed. 3. Does insulin-induced GLUT4 translocation involve sorting of GLUT4 into clathrin-coated vesicles by assembly proteins (APs)? APs interact with other proteins bearing similar sorting motifs as GLUT4, and sort them into clathrin-coated vesicles. These vesicles have been proposed to mediate GLUT4 translocation. The role of APs in GLUT4 trafficking will be investigated by determining if APs interact with GLUT4 and if the interaction is modulated by insulin.

  Website: http://crisp.cit.nih.gov/crisp/Crisp_Query.Generate_Screen

- **Project Title: MECHANISMS OF INSULIN/LH SYNERGY IN THECAL CELLS**

  Principal Investigator & Institution: Veldhuis, Johannes D.; University of Virginia Charlottesville Box 400195 Charlottesville, Va 22904

  Timing: Fiscal Year 2001

  Summary: The **polycystic ovarian syndrome** (PCOS) represents the most common reproductive pathophysiology in pre-menopausal women. Hallmarks of PCOS are increased LH secretion, altered insulin action, and augment ovarian androgen biosynthesis. Overall working hypothesis is that LH and insulin synergize at the level of the ovarian theca cell to drive excessive androgen secretion. Although LH and insulin (or IGF-1) can synergistically amplify ovarian androgen biosynthesis in vivo and by human, hen, rat and pig theca cells in vitro (present data), how LH and insulin collaborate in this fashion is not known. This project will investigate the clinical and molecular mechanisms of IH and insulin synergy in PCOS patients in vivo and on (pig) theca cells in vitro. Our individual aims arise from the following specific hypotheses: I. Preferential suppression of hyperinsulinism (via metformin treatment) of LH hypersecretion (via leuprolide down-regulation) alters the testosterone secretory response to human recombinant LH infusions in PCOS patients; II. In vitro, in pig theca-cell populations, LH and insulin synergistically up-regulate the molecular expression of critical genes that control sterol commitment to androgen biosynthesis; namely, the low-density lipoprotein (LDL) receptor, the steroidogenic acute responsive protein (StAR), and the 17-alpha hydroxylase enzyme; III. In situ, at the single-theca-cell level, LH and insulin synergize by coordinately enhancing multiple sterol-regulatory gene co-expression in individual theca cells; and IV. There are pivotal cis-DNA promoter elements in the StAR and LDL receptor genes that mediate responses to the intracellular signals generated by insulin and LH, acting singly and synergistically. The preceding clinical and basic-science hypotheses and corresponding experiments should help identify novel clinical and molecular mechanisms that govern theca-cell androgen biosynthesis, and thereby offer new insights into the basic pathobiology of PCOS.

Website: http://crisp.cit.nih.gov/crisp/Crisp_Query.Generate_Screen

- **Project Title: NEURAL AND BEHAVIORAL ACTIONS OF ANABOLIC STEROIDS**

Principal Investigator & Institution: Clark, Ann S.; Psychological & Brain Scis; Dartmouth College 11 Rope Ferry Rd. #6210 Hanover, Nh 03755

Timing: Fiscal Year 2001; Project Start 10-DEC-1993; Project End 30-JUN-2004

Summary: (Adapted From The Applicant's Abstract): The long-term objective of this project is to elucidate the neural and behavioral actions of anabolic-androgenic steroid(s) (AAS). Although the majority of published research focuses on males, it has been shown that women and adolescent girls take AAS to improve athletic performance and to achieve a muscular physique. We have demonstrated that individual AAS have discrete and quantifiable effects on the estrous cycle and sexual receptivity in adult rats. The goal of the present proposal is to extend our analysis of AAS effects to include motivation for sexual behavior and to delineate the physiological mechanisms by which AAS affect the nervous system in female rats. First, we will broaden our analysis of AAS effects on female sexual behavior and physiology and address the following questions: (a) does prepubertal AAS administration alter the onset of puberty and produce short- or long-term changes in estrous cyclicity or fertility, (b) do AAS given in combination act synergistically or antagonistically to alter the estrous cycle or sexual behavior, and (c) do AAS alter sexual behaviors that underlie motivation that may be comparable to libido in humans? Second, we will test the role of three brain areas (ventromedial hypothalamus, preoptic area, and lateral septum) rich in androgen and estrogen receptors, in the inhibition of sexual behavior by AAS. Specifically, (a) does direct application of AAS to these brain regions produce effects on behavior that mimic systemic administration, and (b) does the ability of AAS to modulate sexual behaviors at these central sites depend on signaling through steroid (androgen or estrogen) receptors? Third, we will test the possibility that AAS may alter sexual behaviors by acting at gamma-aminobutyric acid type A (GABAa) receptors, because transmission mediated by the GABAergic system is known to modulate sexual behavior. Expressly, does the central administration of AAS modulate sexual behaviors via effects on neuroendocrine processes underlying the AAS modulation of female sexual behavior. Characterizing AAS effects on the central nervous and endocrine systems in laboratory animals will provide valuable scientific evidence that will improve our understanding not only of the physiological and behavioral responses to high dose AAS abuse in women, but also to other naturally occurring disorders that are accompanied by androgen excess, such as **polycystic ovarian syndrome.**

Website: http://crisp.cit.nih.gov/crisp/Crisp_Query.Generate_Screen

- **Project Title: NEURAL CONTRIBUTION TO POLYCYSTIC OVARIAN SYNDROME**

  Principal Investigator & Institution: Ojeda, Sergio R.; Scientist/Division Head; Oregon Health & Science University Portland, or 972393098

  Timing: Fiscal Year 2001

  Summary: The goal of this project was to obtain preliminary evidence for the development of a nonhuman primate model of **polycystic ovarian syndrome** (PCOS). The 4 monkeys used for the experiment had cycled consistently over the previous 12 months (12 or 13 menses recorded, at regular intervals). They were provided with an intraovarian graft of genetically modified baby hamster kidney cells, encapsulated in a polymer of poly [acrylonitrile vinyl chloride, P(AN-VC)]. The surgical implants were performed as close to the first day of the new menses cycle as possible. Two of the monkeys received devices which contained NGF-secreting cells and two of the monkeys received control devices containing unmodified cells. The implants were 0.7 mm outside diameter and 7 mm long. Each monkey received two implants in each ovary. Following laparotomy to expose the ovaries, the implants were inserted into the ovary using a large bore needle and plunger (a suture in the ovarian capsule prevented migration of the device). Following implantation, all four monkeys continued to cycle and did so throughout the six month study; thus, the implants themselves did not affect normal ovarian function. The collected serum samples were assayed for ovarian steroids and luteinizing hormone. Of the steroids analyzed (estradiol, progesterone, testosterone and androstenedione), only androstenedione was elevated following the grafting of NGF producing cells; the other steroids remained constant. Luteinizing hormone levels were also elevated in the monkeys that received the NGF producing grafts. Androstenedione and LH are the two hormones most consistently linked with PCOS in humans. The ovarian morphology following grafting is still being assessed; however, initial observations suggest a possible increase in the number of follicular structures, again reminiscent of PCOS. Although further analysis of the data is necessary, preliminary evaluation suggests that an elevation of intraovarian N GF levels may be one of the components required to generate a nonhuman primate model of PCOS. FUNDING Center-supported project PUBLICATIONS None

  Website: http://crisp.cit.nih.gov/crisp/Crisp_Query.Generate_Screen

- **Project Title: OVARIAN ANDROGEN PRODUCTION AND FOLLICULAR FUNCTION**

  Principal Investigator & Institution: Menon, Jairam K.; Professor; Obstetrics and Gynecology; University of Michigan at Ann Arbor 3003 South State, Room 1040 Ann Arbor, Mi 481091274

  Timing: Fiscal Year 2001; Project Start 01-JUL-2000; Project End 30-JUN-2005

  Summary: The overall goal of this proposal is to examine the molecular basis for the development of hyperandrogenic states and consequent impairment of follicular function. Ovarian hyperandrogenism leads to ovulatory dysfunction including anovulation and infertility. In some cases such as **polycystic ovarian syndrome,** hyperandrogenism usually accompanies increased insulin resistance resulting in elevated insulin levels, and increased IGF-1 system. The altered endocrine and paracrine milieu results in increased androgen production by theca-interstitial cells, ovarian hyperplasia and loss of ovulatory capacity of the follicles. The objective of this proposal is to examine the cellular mechanisms responsible for hyperandrogenism and the resultant effects of excess androgen exposure on follicular function. To accomplish this, three specific aims are proposed. Aim 1 will examine the role of increased cholesterol transport into theca-interstitial cells in response to insulin, IGF-1 and LH. This will be tested by examining the induction of HDL and LDL receptor expression in rat theca-interstitial cells by in situ hypbridization and by Northern blot analysis, and by determining the uptake and utilization of cholesterol for androgen synthesis. Aim 2 will examine the cellular mechanism involved in the deleterious effects of androgen exposure on the ovarian follicular function in response to insulin/IGF-1 and FSH. This will be examined by analyzing changes in cell cycle constituents involved in the progression of restriction points in cell cycle, namely cyclins and cyclin-dependent kinases in response to insul/IGF-1 and FSH in androgen exposed follicles. Aim 3 will examine the effect of androgen exposure on the follicular function. This will be determined by examining the signaling of insulin/IGF-1 and FSH in androgen-exposed follicles. The above studies will be carried out in rat and human tissues. The proposed studies address novel questions central to reproductive endocrinology and are directly relevant to the disorders affecting fertility.

Website: http://crisp.cit.nih.gov/crisp/Crisp_Query.Generate_Screen

- **Project Title: OVARIAN GROWTH FACTORS**

  Principal Investigator & Institution: Hammond, James M.; Professor of Medicine; Medicine; Pennsylvania State Univ Hershey Med Ctr 500 University Dr Hershey, Pa 17033

  Timing: Fiscal Year 2001; Project Start 01-DEC-1996; Project End 30-NOV-2003

  Summary: In the proposed period of support, we will extend our longstanding interest in the ovarian insulin-like growth factor (IGF) system to achieve a level of understanding sufficient to control this system in vivo. Thereafter, the concepts and possibly some of the compounds evaluated can be used to improve fertility in animals and ultimately women. The key to the projected advances is understanding the interface of the IGF-I system with the hormone and growth factor signals during early follicle development and the reproductive cycle. Two control points have been delineated: (1) The physiological control of IGF-I biosynthesis in granulosa cells. In this area, our systems have proven to be uniquely informative. In Specific Aim 1, we will continue these studies to define in molecular terms the interaction of FSH and its cyclic AMP-dependent cascade on the IGF-I promoter. The demonstrated effect of other stimulators of this gene will be tracked to other promoter elements. To test these regulatory principles in vivo, expression IGF-I promoter transgenes will be tested in transgenic mice. (2) In Specific Aim 2, studies of the cell machinery which impacts on the IGF-I gene will be expanded to other aspects of ovarian cell function. The goal of this specific aim is to understand the interaction of IGF with FSH which demonstrably enhances granulosa cell replication, survival and differentiation at various times in the lifespan of the ovarian follicle. These studies will develop a detailed picture of the signal transduction pathways which mediate these effects. Specific Aim 3 employs transgenic approaches to test the hypotheses derived from earlier descriptive studies and in vitro studies in Specific Aims 1 and 2 through transgenic approaches in vivo. The targets for control and investigation will include the local synthesis of IGF-I and IGF-I action mediated through its receptor and multiple points in the phosphorylation cascade which emanate from this receptor. Most of these studies have clinical relevance because inhibitors for the signal cascades to be examined are becoming widely available and because sufficient quantities of various IGF derivatives are now available to use in humans as a possible amplifying mechanism for ovulation. However, the series of experiments of most direct clinical relevance are those which seek to use conditional transgenic technology to build an insulin-resistant model of the **polycystic ovarian syndrome.** If successful, this model could open the door to critical evaluation, understanding, and treatment modalities.

Website: http://crisp.cit.nih.gov/crisp/Crisp_Query.Generate_Screen

- **Project Title: OVARIAN STIMULATION & OOCYTE COMPETENCE IN PRENATALLY ANDROGENIZED FEMALE RHESUS**

    Principal Investigator & Institution: Da, Dumesic; University of Wisconsin Madison 750 University Ave Madison, Wi 53706

    Timing: Fiscal Year 2001

    Summary: OBJECTIVES To determine whether prenatal androgen excess during early gestation in female rhesus monkeys contributes to impaired oocyte developmental competency in adulthood, as part of a study Investigating the origins of increased miscarriage in hyperandrogenic women with **polycystic ovarian syndrome** (PCOS). RESULTS Two prenatally androgenized rhesus monkeys with ovulatory menstrual cycles were stimulated with recombinant human FSH for collection of in vivo matured oocytes. Oocytes were aspirated laparoscopically, and inseminated in vitro following extrusion of the first polar body. Although normal numbers of oocytes were recovered from both monkeys, the proportion of mature (metaphase II) oocytes that were obtained was relatively low (approximately 31%), compared to our long-term average for normal female rhesus monkeys (76%). In one of the prenatally androgenized monkeys (#79135), none of the oocytes completed maturation before 41 hours post hCG, compared to 34 hours for normal female monkeys, and none fertilized, although numerous motile sperm were attached to the zona pellucidae 12 hours after inseminination. In the other prenatally androgenized monkey (#79169), although maturation was quite low, both the incidence of fertilization and development to the blastocyst stage were similar to controls (75% and 65%, respectively). These very preliminary data suggest that oocytes from prenatally androgenized monkeys may be impaired in their ability to mature and to fertilize. FUTURE DIRECTIONS We plan to explore whether oocytes collected from prenatally androgenized monkeys following ovarian stimulation are impaired in their capacity to mature and undergo complete preimplantation development in vitro, to provide novel insight into the high incidence of miscarriage experienced by hyperandrogenic women with PCOS. KEY WORDS oocyte, ovary, **polycystic ovarian syndrome,** androgen excess, miscarriage FUNDING NIH grant RR00167, UW Graduate School Research Committee, UW Medical School Committee

    Website: http://crisp.cit.nih.gov/crisp/Crisp_Query.Generate_Screen

- **Project Title: PATHOPHYSIOLOGIC ROLE OF HYPERINSULINEMIA IN POLYCYSTIC OVARY SYNDROME**

    Principal Investigator & Institution: Chang, R Jeffrey.; Professor & Chairman; University of California San Diego 9500 Gilman Dr, Dept. 0934 La Jolla, Ca 92093

    Timing: Fiscal Year 2001

    Summary: Polycystic ovary syndrome (PCOS) is the most common reproductive-metabolic disorder of women during their child-bearing years affecting 5-10% of this population. The major clinical features include infrequent and irregular menses, excessive hair growth and infertility as result of an ovulation and hyperandrogenism. In recent ears, late age health concerns for these patients have grown largely due to the emergence of insulin resistance and hyperinsulinemia as constitutive components of this disorder. These risks include endometrial cancer, insulin-dependent and noninsulin-dependent diabetes mellitus, hypertension, stroke and cardiovascular disease. Efforts to elucidate the pathogenesis of PCOS have demonstrated distinct abnormalities at each level of the reproductive system as reflected by increased pituitary LH secretion, excessive theca interstitial cell androgen production and arrest of ovarian follicle development. In all of these target tissues insulin had been shown in vitro to enhance cell function, including studies which have utilized both PCOS and normal ovaries. Unfortunately, corresponding in vivo human studies have not been able to corroborate the in vitro results of insulin action. The overall goal of this proposal is to examine in women with PCOS the effect of hyper- insulinemia on the functional capacity of pituitary LH secretion, theca cell androgen production and granulosa cell estrogen production. Our hypothesis is that hyperinsulinemia perpetuates the recognized abnormalities of PCOS by altering these major target tissues. Following baseline studies to determine target tissue responsiveness and sensitivity, PCOS and normal women will have their serum insulin levels raised by the hyperinsulinemic, euglycemic clamp method and the studies will be repeated. Subsequently, subjects will be treated with an insulin enhancing drug, Troglitazone, to reduce hyperinsulinemia after which they will be retested. While on Troglitazone, insulin levels will again be raised and the baseline studies repeated. The results of this vigorous and thorough proposal will allow us to identify in vivo the effects of insulin at each target tissue and determine the clinical impact of hyperinsulinemia on reproductive dysfunction in PCOS.

Website: http://crisp.cit.nih.gov/crisp/Crisp_Query.Generate_Screen

- **Project Title: PILOT--MATHEMATICAL MODELING OF THE MENSTRUAL CYCLE**

    Principal Investigator & Institution: Zeeman, Mary Lou; University of Texas San Antonio San Antonio, Tx 78249

    Timing: Fiscal Year 2003; Project Start 01-AUG-2003; Project End 31-JUL-2006

    Summary: The mathematics of the human menstrual cycle are remarkably understudied. Although several hundred biological papers are written on the topic every year, there is no established mathematical model for the cycle, and there have been only about a dozen mathematical papers addressing the subject in the past 30 years. Almost all of these mathematical papers are over 10 years old, and are thus physiologically out of date. The mathematics of the menstrual cycle is therefore a wide open topic, with a wealth of medical applications, from ovarian and breast cancer, to **polycystic ovarian syndrome,** infertility treatments, and passage to menopause. The long-term goal of this project is to develop a realistic, quantitative model of the neuroendocrine control of the menstrual cycle, in order to make computational predictions about the impact of different hormonal environments on the cycle. We propose to use mathematics, and nonlinear dynamical systems in particular, to analyze the available experimental data in the high dimensional settings required to simultaneously keep track of the hormone interactions at varying time scales. Our approach to the project is three-fold: First: develop physiologically based models of pulsatile LH and GnRH release from populations of secretory cells, mimicking the electrical and chemical communication within and between the cell populations in the hypothalamus and pituitary. Use the GnRH model to drive the LH model while the ovarian hormones modulate the intrinsic frequencies of both models. Analyze the coupled system for transient resonance phenomena modeling the LH surge. Second: generalize the classical work of Lacker et. al. to develop a model of the competitive dynamics among a cohort of ovarian follicles that is consistent with data from normally cycling women; women with infertility conditions such as polycysic ovarian syndrome

(PCO), and women undergoing fertility treatment. Finally: adapt the menstrual cycle model of Selgrade and Schlosser to incorporate these physiological driven sub-models. At each stage of the modeling process we will compare and validate the model with experimental data collected from the literature, experimentalists and fertility clinics.

Website: http://crisp.cit.nih.gov/crisp/Crisp_Query.Generate_Screen

- **Project Title: POLYCYSTIC OVARIAN SYNDROME IN OVERWEIGHT ADOLESCENTS**

  Principal Investigator & Institution: Hoeger, Kathleen M.; Obstetrics and Gynecology; University of Rochester Orpa - Rc Box 270140 Rochester, Ny 14627

  Timing: Fiscal Year 2002; Project Start 01-APR-2002; Project End 31-MAR-2004

  Summary: (provided by applicant): Polycystic Overy Syndrome (PCOS) is a broad-spectrum disease characterized by chronic anovulation and androgen excess, affecting 4-8% of women. Onset of the disorder is recognized to occur around the time of puberty but is often not diagnosed until adulthood. More than half of women with PCOS are obese, and insulin resistance appears to be an important part of its underlying pathophysiology. Long-term consequences in PCOS are now recognized to include increased risk of development of type 2 diabetes mellitus and cardiovascular disease. This has led to an interest in reduction of insulin resistance as a long-term treatment strategy. This reduction in insulin resistance can be accomplished by weight reduction or by insulin sensitizers such as metformin. To date, however, there are limited data on the effectiveness of insulin sensitizers and no data on the impact of weight reduction in adolescents with PCOS. Adolescence is a time of tremendous physical and psychosocial change. Obesity in adolescence is often predictive of lifelong obesity. The constellation of hirsutism, irregular bleeding, and obesity, often seen in adolescents with PCOS, could potentially have lifelong social and health consequences. A successful weight reduction strategy with improvement in insulin sensitivity at the onset of the symptoms of PCOS could have substantial long-term health benefits. The applicant hypothesizes that weight loss and metformin in the overweight adolescent with PCOS can reduce insulin resistance and improve the symptoms and metabolic profile associated with PCOS. Accordingly, a randomized, placebo-controlled, parallel-group trial comparing metformin and intensive lifestyle modification is proposed to gather preliminary data on the rate of ovulation, changes in testosterone and insulin and impact on cardiovascular risk of weight reduction and metformin as compared to placebo in a total of 30 subjects. Data obtained from this pilot trial on recruitment rates, drop-out, compliance, and estimated treatment effect sizes will be used to refine power calculations for a large-scale randomized trial focused on a comparison of metformin and weight reduction in obese adolescents.

  Website: http://crisp.cit.nih.gov/crisp/Crisp_Query.Generate_Screen

- **Project Title: PROGESTERONE/ANDROGEN FEEDBACK CONTROL OF GNRH NEURONS**

  Principal Investigator & Institution: Moenter, Suzanne M.; Associate Professor; University of Virginia Charlottesville Box 400195 Charlottesville, Va 22904

  Timing: Fiscal Year 2003; Project Start 23-APR-2003; Project End 31-MAR-2008

  Summary: Gonadotropin-releasing hormone (GnRH) neurons form the final common pathway regulating reproduction. Pulsatile release of GnRH stimulates secretion of luteinizing hormone (LH) and follicle-stimulating hormone (FSH) from pituitary gonadotropes and is absolutely required for fertility. In female mammals, shifts in

GnRH pulse frequencies help drive the preferential release of LH or FSH at specific times of the cycle to create appropriate hormone milieux for ovarian follicle maturation. GnRH pulse patterns are largely regulated by negative feedback from the ovarian steroids progesterone and estradiol. Although this feedback is well characterized in vivo, the underlying cellular mechanisms and neural pathways have yet to be elucidated. This has precluded understanding the neural components of common forms of hypothalamic infertility, such as **polycystic ovarian syndrome** (PCOS), in which elevated circulating androgen levels are accompanied by a persistent high frequency of LH (and presumably GnRH) release. The latter appears to be due in part to androgens interfering with the efficacy of progesterone feedback. Considerable evidence suggests one mechanism of steroid feedback regulation of GnRH release is transsynaptic. In particular, anatomical and physiological data support a role for gamma-aminobutyric acid (GABA)- and opiate peptide-producing neurons in this communication. Four Specific Aims are proposed to investigate the cellular mechanisms of progesterone feedback, and how androgens might alter the efficacy of progesterone feedback. The primary methodology will be electrophysiological recordings of green-fluorescent protein-identified GnRH neurons in acute brain slices. Aim 1 will investigate the effects of steroid and neurotransmitter milieux on the firing properties and firing patterns of GnRH neurons. Aim 2 will examine how steroids and neurotransmitters alter GABAergic drive to GnRH neurons. Aims 3 and 4 will study the effects of steroids and neurotransmitters on potassium and calcium currents, respectively, as these play major roles in setting firing properties of neurons as well as their ability to respond to synaptic input. These studies will help us understand GnRH neuron physiology in both healthy and diseased states, knowledge paramount for improving treatments for hypothalamic fertility disorders, developing novel contraceptive methods, ensuring effective reproduction in endangered and food-producing species, and understanding other similar neuronal systems.

Website: http://crisp.cit.nih.gov/crisp/Crisp_Query.Generate_Screen

- **Project Title: REGULATION OF FSH ACTION ON PRIMATE OVARY**

    Principal Investigator & Institution: Zeleznick, Anthony; University of Pittsburgh at Pittsburgh 350 Thackeray Hall Pittsburgh, Pa 15260

    Timing: Fiscal Year 2001

    Summary: During the follicular phase of the primate menstrual cycle a single pre-ovulatory follicle is selected to mature and release its oocyte for fertilization and initiation or pregnancy. While it is well established that the gonadotropic hormones follicle stimulating hormone (FSH) and luteinizing hormone (LH) are essential for successful follicular development, over the past decade, it has become evident that other non- gonadotropic factors can also influence ovarian function, either through direct actions on the ovary or by modifying the secretion of FSH and /or LH by the hypothalamic-pituitary axis. In particular, it is clear from a large number of in vitro studies that IGF-I, insulin and androgens play a role in ovarian function by augment (or perhaps inhibiting) the stimulatory actions of FSH and LH on follicular granulosa and theca cells respectively as well as by altering the patterns of FSH and LH secretion. While such actions have been well documented using in vitro approaches, to date their ability to influence the hypothalamic-pituitary-ovarian axis in vivo in primates has not been investigated. Accordingly, we propose to undertake a systematic analysis of the roles of IGF-I, insulin and androgen on the hypothalamic-pituitary-ovarian axis in subhuman primates. In Aim 1 we will test insulin and androgen on the hypothalamic-pituitary-ovarian axis in subhuman primates. In Aim 1 we will test 2, we will test the hypothesis that insulin, IGF-I and androgen influence the sensitivity of the ovarian vivo to FSH. In Aim 2, we will test the hypothesis that insulin, IGF-I and androgen alter the sensitivity of the hypothalamic-pituitary axis to the feedback inhibition of estrogen. In Aim 3 we will test the hypothesis that insulin, IGF-I and androgen alter ovarian cellular proliferation, differentiation and atresia by converging upon intracellular signaling systems that have recently been shown to govern cell proliferation and cell survival. Lastly, in Aim 4, we will determine the effects of insulin, IGF-I and testosterone on menstrual cyclicity in subhuman primates. It is expected that the results of these studies will provide novel information that will have direct bearing not only on normal ovarian function but also pathophysiological aspects of infertility in which normal development of follicles is impaired, especially **polycystic ovarian syndrome** but also pathophysiological aspects of infertility in which normal development of follicles is impaired, especially **polycystic ovarian syndrome** in humans which is associated with alterations in insulin sensitivity and altered androgen production.

Website: http://crisp.cit.nih.gov/crisp/Crisp_Query.Generate_Screen

- **Project Title: REGULATION OF REPRODUCTION**

  Principal Investigator & Institution: Mellon, Synthia H.; Professor; Ob, Gyn and Reproductive Scis; University of California San Francisco 500 Parnassus Ave San Francisco, Ca 94122

  Timing: Fiscal Year 2001; Project Start 01-AUG-1991; Project End 30-JUN-2006

  Summary: The long term objective of this project is a thorough understanding of how steroid hormone synthesis is regulated in a developmental and tissue-specific fashion, and how dysregulation may result in reproductive disorders such as **polycystic ovarian syndrome** (PCOS). The genes for steroidogenic enzymes are transcriptionally regulated at several levels: developmentally, tissue specifically, and hormonally. This regulation shares common features but also differs among the various genes for the steroidogenic enzymes and among various mammals. We will focus on the gene encoding P450c17 (17alpha hydroxylase/17,2 lyase) as it is the key branch point in steroidogenesis, it has been implicated in the etiology of PCOS, and it may be involved in early development of nervous and reproductive systems. Its expression in the human adrenal is required for the synthesis of 17 hydroxy C21 steroids (e.g. cortisol) and for synthesis of C19 sex steroids in the gonads and brain. In the nervous system, expression of P450c17 also results in DHEA synthesis, a potent neuromodulators. We have been using the rodent as our model system for studying the transcriptional regulation of this gene, and have identified cis-acting DNA elements and several novel trans-acting nuclear factors. One of these transcription factors, SET, had been identified from a chromosomal translocation in a patient with acute undifferentiated leukemia, but its role as a transcription factor way unknown. We shall now determine the mechanism of SET action by identifying its DNA binding, transactivation, and potential dimerization domains, and identifying co-factors that may interact with SET to participate in its transactivating functions. AS SET is abundantly expressed and regulates P450c17 expression in the developing gonad and nervous system, we will determine if these co-factors are tissue- specifically expressed, and/or if they modify other known functions of SET. Our studies localizing cis-active elements in the rat P450c17 gene have identified a region bound by a factor that we call StF-IT-2, that interacts with the orphan nuclear receptor SF-1 in a novel way, to regulate P450c17 transcription. We will characterize that interaction, and purify, characterize and clone the cDNA for StF-IT-2. Successful completion of these studies will give us a better understanding of how the gonadal and nervous systems initiate steroidogenesis, the mechanism of action of a new class of transcription factor, novel mechanisms by which SF-1 regulates gene expression, and will identify another transcription factor that may participate in a unique aspect of P450c17 expression.

Website: http://crisp.cit.nih.gov/crisp/Crisp_Query.Generate_Screen

- **Project Title: REPRODUCTIVE CONSEQUENCES OF PRENATAL ANDROGENIZATION**

   Principal Investigator & Institution: Padmanabhan, Vasantha; Professor of Pediatrics; Pediatrics & Communicable Dis; University of Michigan at Ann Arbor 3003 South State, Room 1040 Ann Arbor, Mi 481091274

   Timing: Fiscal Year 2001; Project Start 08-AUG-2001; Project End 31-MAY-2006

   Summary: Polycystic ovarian syndrome (PCOS) is the most common endocrinopathy and it affects 10 percent of reproductive-aged women. The etiology of chronic hyperandrogenic anovulations, such as PCOS, may have genetic underpinnings. Although the underlying mechanisms are unknown, PCOS is now recognized as hyperandrogenism accompanied by anovulation. Polycystic ovarian morphology is highly correlated with conditions in which the fetus has been exposed to high amounts of sex steroids before birth. For example, women with classical 21-hydroxylase deficiency mimic PCOS, exhibit anovulation, ovarian hyperandrogenism, and LH hypersecretion. Perhaps excess sex steroids early in life may provide a hormonal "insult" that results in manifestation of PCOS later in adulthood. This proposal aims to use a new model, the prenatally-androgenized sheep (long gestation, mono-ovular species), to investigate causal mechanisms for the developmental origins of PCOS. Our preliminary studies indicate that these sheep develop ovulatory defects during adulthood similar to those of women with PCOS: anovulation, elevated LH levels, hyperandrogenemia, hyperinsulinemia, and multifollicular ovaries. In this proposal, we will test the following hypothesis: prenatal exposure to androgens disrupts adult reproductive function culminating in hyperandrogenic anovulation and that this disruption is mediated via reduced sensitivity to the positive feedback actions of estradiol, abnormal gonadotropic drive and/or altered ovarian sensitivity to FSH. The specific Aims of the proposed research are to determine 1) the extent to which fetal exposure to androgens disrupts reproductive cyclicity, ovarian function, ovulatory capacity and fertility in adulthood, (2) if reduced sensitivity to estradiol stimulatory feedback of gonadotropin secretion contributes to the disruptive effects of prenatal- androgenization on postnatal reproductive cyclicity, and (3) if abnormal gonadotropic drive and/or reduced ovarian sensitivity to FSH contributes to the disruptive effects of prenatal- androgenization on postnatal reproductive cyclicity. If our hypothesis proves to be correct, this would form the basis for a distinct developmental origin of an important reproductive disease in adulthood. Specifically it will establish that discrete, experimentally induced androgen excess of fetal sheep provides the first clear etiology for hyperandrogenic anovulation in adulthood.

   Website: http://crisp.cit.nih.gov/crisp/Crisp_Query.Generate_Screen

- **Project Title: SAFETY AND EFFICACY OF TROGLITAZONE IN POLYCYSTIC OVARIAN SYNDROME**

   Principal Investigator & Institution: Meyer, William R.; University of North Carolina Chapel Hill Office of Sponsored Research Chapel Hill, Nc 27599

   Timing: Fiscal Year 2001

   Summary: This abstract is not available.

Website: http://crisp.cit.nih.gov/crisp/Crisp_Query.Generate_Screen

- **Project Title:** TRANSCRIPTIONAL REGULATION OF LH BETA GENE EXPRESSION

    Principal Investigator & Institution: Halvorson, Lisa M.; New England Medical Center Hospitals 750 Washington St Boston, Ma 021111533

    Timing: Fiscal Year 2001; Project Start 01-JUL-1999; Project End 30-JUN-2004

    Summary: The pituitary gonadotropins, luteinizing hormone (LH) and follicle-stimulating hormone (FSH), are critical modulators of gamete maturation and gonadal steroidogenesis. Recent evidence has demonstrated that the transcription factors, steroidogenic factor-1 (SF-1) and early growth response gene 1 (Egr-1), regulate expression of the LHbeta-subunit gene. The long-term objective of our work is to understand fully the transcription factors and cis-elements which modulate LHbeta gene expression, information which will provide insight into both normal and abnormal reproductive function. The Specific Aims of this proposal are: 1) to characterize the role of the bicoid-related transcription factor, Ptx1, in mediating tissue-specific LHbeta gene expression, 2) to define the physiologic importance of the LHbeta-Ptx1 cis-element(s) in primary gonadotropes in culture and in vivo, and 3) to identify the molecular mechanisms which mediate cAMP/PKA-induced stimulation of LHbeta gene promoter activity. In Aim 1, based on a report by Drouin and co-workers, we hypothesize that Ptx1 acts alone and in synergy with SF-1 to increase LHbeta promoter activity, as will be tested by electrophoretic mobility shift assay, transient transfection of immortalized cell lines, and generation of Ptx1 "knockdown" cell lines. In Aim 2A, primary pituitary cell cultures will be infected using a highly efficient, recombinant adenovirus approach in order to define the 5'flanking region which confers gonadotrope-specific expression. The defined gonadotrope-specific region will then be used in reporter constructs as either the wild-type sequence or with a mutation in the Ptx1-site(s) identified in Aim 1. We predict that the presence of a mutation in the Ptx1 site(s) will markedly blunt reporter expression in both cultured primary pituitary cells (Aim 2B) and transgenic mouse lines (Aim 2C), verifying the physiologic importance of Ptx1 to LHbeta gene expression. In Aim 3, we propose to test the hypothesis that cAMP/PKA-induced increases in LHbeta promoter activity are due to: A) PKA-regulated changes in SF-1 and/or Egr-1 gene expression or post-translational modifications, and/or B) putative AP-2 cis-element(s) in the LHbeta gene promoter sequence. By further characterizing factors which mediate tissue-specific and hormonally-regulated LHbeta gene expression, these studies will contribute to our understanding of normal reproductive physiology, as well as the pathophysiology of disorders including infertility, **polycystic ovarian syndrome,** hypothalamic hypogonadism, and premature and delayed puberty.

    Website: http://crisp.cit.nih.gov/crisp/Crisp_Query.Generate_Screen

E-Journals: PubMed Central[3]

PubMed Central (PMC) is a digital archive of life sciences journal literature developed and managed by the National Center for Biotechnology Information (NCBI) at the U.S. National Library of Medicine (NLM).[4] Access to this growing archive of e-journals is free and

---

[3] Adapted from the National Library of Medicine: **http://www.pubmedcentral.nih.gov/about/intro.html**.

[4] With PubMed Central, NCBI is taking the lead in preservation and maintenance of open access to electronic literature, just as NLM has done for decades with printed biomedical literature. PubMed Central aims to become a world-class library of the digital age.

unrestricted.[5] To search, go to **http://www.ncbi.nlm.nih.gov/entrez/query.fcgi?db=Pmc**, and type "polycystic ovarian syndrome" (or synonyms) into the search box. This search gives you access to full-text articles. The following is a sample of items found for polycystic ovarian syndrome in the PubMed Central database:

- **A paradigm for finding genes for a complex human trait: Polycystic ovary syndrome and follistatin.** by Odunsi K, Kidd KK.; 1999 Jul 20; http://www.pubmedcentral.gov/articlerender.fcgi?tool=pmcentrez&artid=33617

- **Evidence for a genetic basis for hyperandrogenemia in polycystic ovary syndrome.** by Legro RS, Driscoll D, Strauss JF III, Fox J, Dunaif A.; 1998 Dec 8; http://www.pubmedcentral.gov/articlerender.fcgi?tool=pmcentrez&artid=24557

- **Metformin in polycystic ovary syndrome: systematic review and meta-analysis.** by Lord JM, Flight IH, Norman RJ.; 2003 Oct 25; http://www.pubmedcentral.gov/articlerender.fcgi?tool=pmcentrez&artid=259161

- **Molecular Basis of Aromatase Deficiency in an Adult Female with Sexual Infantilism and Polycystic Ovaries.** by Ito Y, Fisher CR, Conte FA, Grumbach MM, Simpson ER.; 1993 Dec 15; http://www.pubmedcentral.gov/articlerender.fcgi?tool=pmcentrez&rendertype=abstract&artid=48046

- **Serine Phosphorylation of Human P450c17 Increases 17,20-Lyase Activity: Implications for Adrenarche and the Polycystic Ovary Syndrome.** by Zhang L, Rodriguez H, Ohno S, Miller WL.; 1995 Nov 7; http://www.pubmedcentral.gov/articlerender.fcgi?tool=pmcentrez&rendertype=abstract&artid=40663

- **Thirty-seven candidate genes for polycystic ovary syndrome: Strongest evidence for linkage is with follistatin.** by Urbanek M, Legro RS, Driscoll DA, Azziz R, Ehrmann DA, Norman RJ, Strauss JF III, Spielman RS, Dunaif A.; 1999 Jul 20; http://www.pubmedcentral.gov/articlerender.fcgi?tool=pmcentrez&artid=17558

The National Library of Medicine: PubMed

One of the quickest and most comprehensive ways to find academic studies in both English and other languages is to use PubMed, maintained by the National Library of Medicine.[6] The advantage of PubMed over previously mentioned sources is that it covers a greater number of domestic and foreign references. It is also free to use. If the publisher has a Web site that offers full text of its journals, PubMed will provide links to that site, as well as to sites offering other related data. User registration, a subscription fee, or some other type of fee may be required to access the full text of articles in some journals.

To generate your own bibliography of studies dealing with polycystic ovarian syndrome, simply go to the PubMed Web site at **http://www.ncbi.nlm.nih.gov/pubmed**. Type

---

[5] The value of PubMed Central, in addition to its role as an archive, lies in the availability of data from diverse sources stored in a common format in a single repository. Many journals already have online publishing operations, and there is a growing tendency to publish material online only, to the exclusion of print.

[6] PubMed was developed by the National Center for Biotechnology Information (NCBI) at the National Library of Medicine (NLM) at the National Institutes of Health (NIH). The PubMed database was developed in conjunction with publishers of biomedical literature as a search tool for accessing literature citations and linking to full-text journal articles at Web sites of participating publishers. Publishers that participate in PubMed supply NLM with their citations electronically prior to or at the time of publication.

"polycystic ovarian syndrome" (or synonyms) into the search box, and click "Go." The following is the type of output you can expect from PubMed for polycystic ovarian syndrome (hyperlinks lead to article summaries):

- **A comparative, randomized study of low-dose human menopausal gonadotropin and follicle-stimulating hormone in women with polycystic ovarian syndrome.**
  Author(s): Sagle MA, Hamilton-Fairley D, Kiddy DS, Franks S.
  Source: Fertility and Sterility. 1991 January; 55(1): 56-60.
  http://www.ncbi.nlm.nih.gov:80/entrez/query.fcgi?cmd=Retrieve&db=PubMed&list_uids=1898891&dopt=Abstract

- **A pilot study of the long-term effects of acipimox in polycystic ovarian syndrome.**
  Author(s): Ciampelli M, Leoni F, Lattanzi F, Guido M, Apa R, Lanzone A.
  Source: Human Reproduction (Oxford, England). 2002 March; 17(3): 647-53.
  http://www.ncbi.nlm.nih.gov:80/entrez/query.fcgi?cmd=Retrieve&db=PubMed&list_uids=11870117&dopt=Abstract

- **A possible approach to the treatment of polycystic ovarian syndrome using focused ultrasound.**
  Author(s): Moussatov AG, Baker AC, Duck FA.
  Source: Ultrasonics. 1998 July; 36(8): 893-900.
  http://www.ncbi.nlm.nih.gov:80/entrez/query.fcgi?cmd=Retrieve&db=PubMed&list_uids=9695768&dopt=Abstract

- **A preponderance of basic luteinizing hormone (LH) isoforms accompanies inappropriate hypersecretion of both basal and pulsatile LH in adolescents with polycystic ovarian syndrome.**
  Author(s): Ropelato MG, Garcia-Rudaz MC, Castro-Fernandez C, Ulloa-Aguirre A, Escobar ME, Barontini M, Veldhuis JD.
  Source: The Journal of Clinical Endocrinology and Metabolism. 1999 December; 84(12): 4629-36.
  http://www.ncbi.nlm.nih.gov:80/entrez/query.fcgi?cmd=Retrieve&db=PubMed&list_uids=10599730&dopt=Abstract

- **A putative relationship between valproic acid and polycystic ovarian syndrome: implications for treatment of women with seizure and bipolar disorders.**
  Author(s): Joffe H, Hall JE, Cohen LS, Taylor AE, Baldessarini RJ.
  Source: Harvard Review of Psychiatry. 2003 March-April; 11(2): 99-108. Review.
  http://www.ncbi.nlm.nih.gov:80/entrez/query.fcgi?cmd=Retrieve&db=PubMed&list_uids=12868510&dopt=Abstract

- **A simple treatment for polycystic ovarian syndrome.**
  Author(s): Gjonnaess H.
  Source: World Health Forum. 1990; 11(2): 214-7.
  http://www.ncbi.nlm.nih.gov:80/entrez/query.fcgi?cmd=Retrieve&db=PubMed&list_uids=2148677&dopt=Abstract

- **A specific elevation in tissue plasminogen activator antigen in women with polycystic ovarian syndrome.**
  Author(s): Kelly CJ, Lyall H, Petrie JR, Gould GW, Connell JM, Rumley A, Lowe GD, Sattar N.
  Source: The Journal of Clinical Endocrinology and Metabolism. 2002 July; 87(7): 3287-90.
  http://www.ncbi.nlm.nih.gov:80/entrez/query.fcgi?cmd=Retrieve&db=PubMed&list_uids=12107238&dopt=Abstract

- **Abnormal luteinizing hormone response patterns to synthetic gonadotrophin releasing hormone in patients with polycystic ovarian syndrome.**
  Author(s): Katz M, Carr PJ.
  Source: The Journal of Endocrinology. 1976 August; 70(2): 163-71.
  http://www.ncbi.nlm.nih.gov:80/entrez/query.fcgi?cmd=Retrieve&db=PubMed&list_uids=787466&dopt=Abstract

- **Accelerated 24-hour luteinizing hormone pulsatile activity in adolescent girls with ovarian hyperandrogenism: relevance to the developmental phase of polycystic ovarian syndrome.**
  Author(s): Apter D, Butzow T, Laughlin GA, Yen SS.
  Source: The Journal of Clinical Endocrinology and Metabolism. 1994 July; 79(1): 119-25.
  http://www.ncbi.nlm.nih.gov:80/entrez/query.fcgi?cmd=Retrieve&db=PubMed&list_uids=8027216&dopt=Abstract

- **Acth function in women with the polycystic ovarian syndrome.**
  Author(s): Horrocks PM, Kandeel FR, London DR, Butt WR, Lynch SS, Holder G, Logan-Edwards R.
  Source: Clinical Endocrinology. 1983 August; 19(2): 143-50.
  http://www.ncbi.nlm.nih.gov:80/entrez/query.fcgi?cmd=Retrieve&db=PubMed&list_uids=6309433&dopt=Abstract

- **Acute pituitary-ovarian response during chronic luteinizing hormone-releasing hormone agonist administration in polycystic ovarian syndrome.**
  Author(s): Faure N, Lemay A.
  Source: Clinical Endocrinology. 1988 October; 29(4): 403-10.
  http://www.ncbi.nlm.nih.gov:80/entrez/query.fcgi?cmd=Retrieve&db=PubMed&list_uids=3150825&dopt=Abstract

- **Adhesion formation after laparoscopic ovarian cautery for polycystic ovarian syndrome: lack of correlation with pregnancy rate.**
  Author(s): Greenblatt EM, Casper RF.
  Source: Fertility and Sterility. 1993 November; 60(5): 766-70.
  http://www.ncbi.nlm.nih.gov:80/entrez/query.fcgi?cmd=Retrieve&db=PubMed&list_uids=8224258&dopt=Abstract

- **Adhesion formation after ovarian electrocauterization on patients with polycystic ovarian syndrome.**
  Author(s): Dabirashrafi H, Mohamad K, Behjatnia Y, Moghadami-Tabrizi N.
  Source: Fertility and Sterility. 1991 June; 55(6): 1200-1.
  http://www.ncbi.nlm.nih.gov:80/entrez/query.fcgi?cmd=Retrieve&db=PubMed&list_uids=2037115&dopt=Abstract

- **Adipocyte insulin action following ovulation in polycystic ovarian syndrome.**
  Author(s): Marsden PJ, Murdoch AP, Taylor R.
  Source: Human Reproduction (Oxford, England). 1999 September; 14(9): 2216-22.
  http://www.ncbi.nlm.nih.gov:80/entrez/query.fcgi?cmd=Retrieve&db=PubMed&list_uids=10469683&dopt=Abstract

- **Age and follicular phase estradiol are better predictors of pregnancy outcome than luteinizing hormone in menotropin ovulation induction for anovulatory polycystic ovarian syndrome.**
  Author(s): McClure N, McDonald J, Kovacs GT, Healy DL, McCloud PI, McQuinn B, Burger HG.
  Source: Fertility and Sterility. 1993 April; 59(4): 729-33.
  http://www.ncbi.nlm.nih.gov:80/entrez/query.fcgi?cmd=Retrieve&db=PubMed&list_uids=8458487&dopt=Abstract

- **Alterations in cardiac flow parameters in patients with polycystic ovarian syndrome.**
  Author(s): Tiras MB, Yalcin R, Noyan V, Maral I, Yildirim M, Dortlemez O, Daya S.
  Source: Human Reproduction (Oxford, England). 1999 August; 14(8): 1949-52.
  http://www.ncbi.nlm.nih.gov:80/entrez/query.fcgi?cmd=Retrieve&db=PubMed&list_uids=10438405&dopt=Abstract

- **An overview of the diagnostic considerations in polycystic ovarian syndrome.**
  Author(s): Crowley WF Jr, Hall JE, Martin KA, Adams J, Taylor AE.
  Source: Annals of the New York Academy of Sciences. 1993 May 28; 687: 235-41.
  http://www.ncbi.nlm.nih.gov:80/entrez/query.fcgi?cmd=Retrieve&db=PubMed&list_uids=8323178&dopt=Abstract

- **Androgen hyperfunction and excessive heterosexual hair growth in women, with special attention to the polycystic ovarian syndrome.**
  Author(s): Lunde O.
  Source: Acta Obstetricia Et Gynecologica Scandinavica. 1991; 70(4-5): 395-6.
  http://www.ncbi.nlm.nih.gov:80/entrez/query.fcgi?cmd=Retrieve&db=PubMed&list_uids=1746274&dopt=Abstract

- **Androgen response in polycystic ovarian syndrome to FSH treatment after LHRH agonist suppression.**
  Author(s): Hamori M, Zwirner M, Cledon P, Tinneberg HR.
  Source: Int J Fertil. 1992 May-June; 37(3): 171-5.
  http://www.ncbi.nlm.nih.gov:80/entrez/query.fcgi?cmd=Retrieve&db=PubMed&list_uids=1355764&dopt=Abstract

- **Androgen sulfate and glucuronide conjugates in nonhirsute and hirsute women with polycystic ovarian syndrome.**
  Author(s): Matteri RK, Stanczyk FZ, Gentzschein EE, Delgado C, Lobo RA.
  Source: American Journal of Obstetrics and Gynecology. 1989 December; 161(6 Pt 1): 1704-9.
  http://www.ncbi.nlm.nih.gov:80/entrez/query.fcgi?cmd=Retrieve&db=PubMed&list_uids=2532471&dopt=Abstract

- **Androgens in polycystic ovarian syndrome.**
  Author(s): Pugeat M, Nicolas MH, Craves JC, Alvarado-Dubost C, Fimbel S, Dechaud H, Lejeune H.
  Source: Annals of the New York Academy of Sciences. 1993 May 28; 687: 124-35. Review.
  http://www.ncbi.nlm.nih.gov:80/entrez/query.fcgi?cmd=Retrieve&db=PubMed&list_uids=8323167&dopt=Abstract

- **Assessment of ovaries by magnetic resonance imaging in patients presenting with polycystic ovarian syndrome.**
  Author(s): Faure N, Prat X, Bastide A, Lemay A.
  Source: Human Reproduction (Oxford, England). 1989 May; 4(4): 468-72.
  http://www.ncbi.nlm.nih.gov:80/entrez/query.fcgi?cmd=Retrieve&db=PubMed&list_uids=2501338&dopt=Abstract

- **Assisted reproduction techniques in polycystic ovarian syndrome.**
  Author(s): Tarlatzis BC, Grimbizis G.
  Source: Annals of the New York Academy of Sciences. 1993 May 28; 687: 280-7. Review.
  http://www.ncbi.nlm.nih.gov:80/entrez/query.fcgi?cmd=Retrieve&db=PubMed&list_uids=8323183&dopt=Abstract

- **Benefits of continuous physiological pulsatile gonadotropin-releasing hormone therapy in women with polycystic ovarian syndrome.**
  Author(s): Corenthal L, Von Hagen S, Larkins D, Ibrahim J, Santoro N.
  Source: Fertility and Sterility. 1994 June; 61(6): 1027-33.
  http://www.ncbi.nlm.nih.gov:80/entrez/query.fcgi?cmd=Retrieve&db=PubMed&list_uids=8194612&dopt=Abstract

- **Body composition and regional fat distribution in polycystic ovarian syndrome. Relationship to hormonal and metabolic profiles.**
  Author(s): Bringer J, Lefebvre P, Boulet F, Grigorescu F, Renard E, Hedon B, Orsetti A, Jaffiol C.
  Source: Annals of the New York Academy of Sciences. 1993 May 28; 687: 115-23.
  http://www.ncbi.nlm.nih.gov:80/entrez/query.fcgi?cmd=Retrieve&db=PubMed&list_uids=8323166&dopt=Abstract

- **Body weight, body mass index, and age: predictors of menotropin dose and cycle outcome in polycystic ovarian syndrome?**
  Author(s): McClure N, McQuinn B, McDonald J, Kovacs GT, Healy DL, Burger HG.
  Source: Fertility and Sterility. 1992 September; 58(3): 622-4.
  http://www.ncbi.nlm.nih.gov:80/entrez/query.fcgi?cmd=Retrieve&db=PubMed&list_uids=1521660&dopt=Abstract

- **Body weight, hyperinsulinemia, and gonadotropin levels in the polycystic ovarian syndrome: evidence of two distinct populations.**
  Author(s): Dale PO, Tanbo T, Vaaler S, Abyholm T.
  Source: Fertility and Sterility. 1992 September; 58(3): 487-91.
  http://www.ncbi.nlm.nih.gov:80/entrez/query.fcgi?cmd=Retrieve&db=PubMed&list_uids=1521640&dopt=Abstract

- **Bulimia and polycystic ovarian syndrome?**
  Author(s): Chapdelaine PA Jr.
  Source: Fertility and Sterility. 1991 September; 56(3): 585-6.
  http://www.ncbi.nlm.nih.gov:80/entrez/query.fcgi?cmd=Retrieve&db=PubMed&list_uids=1894042&dopt=Abstract

- **Bulimic eating patterns should be stabilised in polycystic ovarian syndrome.**
  Author(s): Morgan JF.
  Source: Bmj (Clinical Research Ed.). 1999 January 30; 318(7179): 328.
  http://www.ncbi.nlm.nih.gov:80/entrez/query.fcgi?cmd=Retrieve&db=PubMed&list_uids=9924069&dopt=Abstract

- **Can women with gonadotropin levels diagnostic of polycystic ovarian syndrome benefit from therapy with dopamine agonists?**
  Author(s): Harrison RF, Synnott M, O'Moore R, O'Moore M.
  Source: Annals of the New York Academy of Sciences. 1993 May 28; 687: 272-9.
  http://www.ncbi.nlm.nih.gov:80/entrez/query.fcgi?cmd=Retrieve&db=PubMed&list_uids=8100697&dopt=Abstract

- **Cardiovascular risk in women with polycystic ovarian syndrome.**
  Author(s): Guzick DS.
  Source: Semin Reprod Endocrinol. 1996 February; 14(1): 45-9. Review. No Abstract Available.
  http://www.ncbi.nlm.nih.gov:80/entrez/query.fcgi?cmd=Retrieve&db=PubMed&list_uids=8796926&dopt=Abstract

- **Cellular mechanisms of insulin resistance in polycystic ovarian syndrome.**
  Author(s): Ciaraldi TP, el-Roeiy A, Madar Z, Reichart D, Olefsky JM, Yen SS.
  Source: The Journal of Clinical Endocrinology and Metabolism. 1992 August; 75(2): 577-83.
  http://www.ncbi.nlm.nih.gov:80/entrez/query.fcgi?cmd=Retrieve&db=PubMed&list_uids=1322430&dopt=Abstract

- **Central retinal vein occlusion associated with the polycystic ovarian syndrome.**
  Author(s): Salzmann J, Jagger J.
  Source: Int J Clin Pract. 1997 July-August; 51(5): 339-41.
  http://www.ncbi.nlm.nih.gov:80/entrez/query.fcgi?cmd=Retrieve&db=PubMed&list_uids=9489102&dopt=Abstract

- **Changes in luteinizing hormone and insulin secretion in polycystic ovarian syndrome.**
  Author(s): Fulghesu AM, Cucinelli F, Pavone V, Murgia F, Guido M, Caruso A, Mancuso S, Lanzone A.
  Source: Human Reproduction (Oxford, England). 1999 March; 14(3): 611-7.
  http://www.ncbi.nlm.nih.gov:80/entrez/query.fcgi?cmd=Retrieve&db=PubMed&list_uids=10221684&dopt=Abstract

- **Changes of bioactive luteinizing hormone after laparoscopic ovarian cautery in patients with polycystic ovarian syndrome.**
  Author(s): Sakata M, Tasaka K, Kurachi H, Terakawa N, Miyake A, Tanizawa O.
  Source: Fertility and Sterility. 1990 April; 53(4): 610-3.
  http://www.ncbi.nlm.nih.gov:80/entrez/query.fcgi?cmd=Retrieve&db=PubMed&list_uids=2138570&dopt=Abstract

- **Characteristics predictive of response to ovarian diathermy in women with polycystic ovarian syndrome.**
  Author(s): Stegmann BJ, Craig HR, Bay RC, Coonrod DV, Brady MJ, Garbaciak JA Jr.
  Source: American Journal of Obstetrics and Gynecology. 2003 May; 188(5): 1171-3.
  http://www.ncbi.nlm.nih.gov:80/entrez/query.fcgi?cmd=Retrieve&db=PubMed&list_uids=12748468&dopt=Abstract

- **Characterization of intrafollicular steroid hormones, inhibin, and follistatin in women with and without polycystic ovarian syndrome following gonadotropin hyperstimulation.**
  Author(s): Lambert-Messerlian G, Taylor A, Leykin L, Isaacson K, Toth T, Chang Y, Schneyer A.
  Source: Biology of Reproduction. 1997 November; 57(5): 1211-6.
  http://www.ncbi.nlm.nih.gov:80/entrez/query.fcgi?cmd=Retrieve&db=PubMed&list_uids=9369189&dopt=Abstract

- **Choice of stimulation in polycystic ovarian syndrome: the influence of obesity.**
  Author(s): Galtier-Dereure F, Pujol P, Dewailly D, Bringer J.
  Source: Human Reproduction (Oxford, England). 1997 October; 12 Suppl 1: 88-96. Review.
  http://www.ncbi.nlm.nih.gov:80/entrez/query.fcgi?cmd=Retrieve&db=PubMed&list_uids=9403325&dopt=Abstract

- **Circulating and ovarian IGF binding proteins: potential roles in normo-ovulatory cycles and in polycystic ovarian syndrome.**
  Author(s): Giudice LC, van Dessel HJ, Cataldo NA, Chandrasekher YA, Yap OW, Fauser BC.
  Source: Progress in Growth Factor Research. 1995; 6(2-4): 397-408. Review.
  http://www.ncbi.nlm.nih.gov:80/entrez/query.fcgi?cmd=Retrieve&db=PubMed&list_uids=8817683&dopt=Abstract

- **Circulating follistatin concentrations are higher and activin concentrations are lower in polycystic ovarian syndrome.**
  Author(s): Norman RJ, Milner CR, Groome NP, Robertson DM.
  Source: Human Reproduction (Oxford, England). 2001 April; 16(4): 668-72.
  http://www.ncbi.nlm.nih.gov:80/entrez/query.fcgi?cmd=Retrieve&db=PubMed&list_uids=11278215&dopt=Abstract

- **Clinical, endocrine and metabolic effects of metformin added to ethinyl estradiol-cyproterone acetate in non-obese women with polycystic ovarian syndrome: a randomized controlled study.**
  Author(s): Elter K, Imir G, Durmusoglu F.
  Source: Human Reproduction (Oxford, England). 2002 July; 17(7): 1729-37.
  http://www.ncbi.nlm.nih.gov:80/entrez/query.fcgi?cmd=Retrieve&db=PubMed&list_uids=12093831&dopt=Abstract

- **Clomiphene citrate increases insulin-like growth factor binding protein-1 and reduces insulin-like growth factor-I without correcting insulin resistance associated with polycystic ovarian syndrome.**
  Author(s): de Leo V, la Marca A, Morgante G, Ciotta L, Mencaglia L, Cianci A, Petraglia F.
  Source: Human Reproduction (Oxford, England). 2000 November; 15(11): 2302-5.
  http://www.ncbi.nlm.nih.gov:80/entrez/query.fcgi?cmd=Retrieve&db=PubMed&list_uids=11056123&dopt=Abstract

- **Co-administration of metformin during rFSH treatment in patients with clomiphene citrate-resistant polycystic ovarian syndrome: a prospective randomized trial.**
  Author(s): Yarali H, Yildiz BO, Demirol A, Zeyneloglu HB, Yigit N, Bukulmez O, Koray Z.
  Source: Human Reproduction (Oxford, England). 2002 February; 17(2): 289-94.
  http://www.ncbi.nlm.nih.gov:80/entrez/query.fcgi?cmd=Retrieve&db=PubMed&list_uids=11821265&dopt=Abstract

- **Common treatment of polycystic ovarian syndrome and major depressive disorder: case report and review.**
  Author(s): Rasgon NL, Carter MS, Elman S, Bauer M, Love M, Korenman SG.
  Source: Current Drug Targets. Immune, Endocrine and Metabolic Disorders. 2002 April; 2(1): 97-102. Review.
  http://www.ncbi.nlm.nih.gov:80/entrez/query.fcgi?cmd=Retrieve&db=PubMed&list_uids=12477299&dopt=Abstract

- **Comparison of urinary human follicle-stimulating hormone and human menopausal gonadotropin for ovarian stimulation in polycystic ovarian syndrome.**
  Author(s): Larsen T, Larsen JF, Schioler V, Bostofte E, Felding C.
  Source: Fertility and Sterility. 1990 March; 53(3): 426-31.
  http://www.ncbi.nlm.nih.gov:80/entrez/query.fcgi?cmd=Retrieve&db=PubMed&list_uids=2106449&dopt=Abstract

- **Correction of hyperandrogenemia by laparoscopic ovarian cautery in women with polycystic ovarian syndrome is not accompanied by improved insulin sensitivity or lipid-lipoprotein levels.**
  Author(s): Lemieux S, Lewis GF, Ben-Chetrit A, Steiner G, Greenblatt EM.
  Source: The Journal of Clinical Endocrinology and Metabolism. 1999 November; 84(11): 4278-82.
  http://www.ncbi.nlm.nih.gov:80/entrez/query.fcgi?cmd=Retrieve&db=PubMed&list_uids=10566685&dopt=Abstract

- **Diagnostic dilemmas in polycystic ovarian syndrome.**
  Author(s): Batrinos ML.
  Source: Annals of the New York Academy of Sciences. 1993 May 28; 687: 230-4. Review.
  http://www.ncbi.nlm.nih.gov:80/entrez/query.fcgi?cmd=Retrieve&db=PubMed&list_uids=8323177&dopt=Abstract

- **Different responses of insulin, C-peptide, and testosterone to an oral glucose tolerance test in two groups of women with polycystic ovarian syndrome.**
  Author(s): Ke WX, Shan GQ, Hua SY.
  Source: Acta Obstetricia Et Gynecologica Scandinavica. 1996 February; 75(2): 166-9.
  http://www.ncbi.nlm.nih.gov:80/entrez/query.fcgi?cmd=Retrieve&db=PubMed&list_uids=8604605&dopt=Abstract

- **Differential androgen response to adrenocorticotrophin hormone stimulation and effect of opioid antagonist on insulin secretion in polycystic ovarian syndrome.**
  Author(s): Lanzone A, Fulghesu AM, Guido M, Ciampelli M, Caruso A, Mancuso S.
  Source: Human Reproduction (Oxford, England). 1994 December; 9(12): 2242-6.
  http://www.ncbi.nlm.nih.gov:80/entrez/query.fcgi?cmd=Retrieve&db=PubMed&list_uids=7714138&dopt=Abstract

- **Differential androgen response to adrenocorticotropic hormone stimulation in polycystic ovarian syndrome: relationship with insulin secretion.**
  Author(s): Lanzone A, Fulghesu AM, Guido M, Fortini A, Caruso A, Mancuso S.
  Source: Fertility and Sterility. 1992 August; 58(2): 296-301.
  http://www.ncbi.nlm.nih.gov:80/entrez/query.fcgi?cmd=Retrieve&db=PubMed&list_uids=1321739&dopt=Abstract

- **Disruption of the joint synchrony of luteinizing hormone, testosterone, and androstenedione secretion in adolescents with polycystic ovarian syndrome.**
  Author(s): Veldhuis JD, Pincus SM, Garcia-Rudaz MC, Ropelato MG, Escobar ME, Barontini M.
  Source: The Journal of Clinical Endocrinology and Metabolism. 2001 January; 86(1): 72-9.
  http://www.ncbi.nlm.nih.gov:80/entrez/query.fcgi?cmd=Retrieve&db=PubMed&list_uids=11231981&dopt=Abstract

- **Disruption of the synchronous secretion of leptin, LH, and ovarian androgens in nonobese adolescents with the polycystic ovarian syndrome.**
  Author(s): Veldhuis JD, Pincus SM, Garcia-Rudaz MC, Ropelato MG, Escobar ME, Barontini M.
  Source: The Journal of Clinical Endocrinology and Metabolism. 2001 August; 86(8): 3772-8.
  http://www.ncbi.nlm.nih.gov:80/entrez/query.fcgi?cmd=Retrieve&db=PubMed&list_uids=11502810&dopt=Abstract

- **Does laparoscopic ovarian diathermy affect the outcome of IVF-embryo transfer in women with polycystic ovarian syndrome? A retrospective comparative study.**
  Author(s): Tozer AJ, Al-Shawaf T, Zosmer A, Hussain S, Wilson C, Lower AM, Grudzinskas JG.
  Source: Human Reproduction (Oxford, England). 2001 January; 16(1): 91-95.
  http://www.ncbi.nlm.nih.gov:80/entrez/query.fcgi?cmd=Retrieve&db=PubMed&list_uids=11139543&dopt=Abstract

- **Does obesity diminish the positive effect of oral contraceptive treatment on hyperandrogenism in women with polycystic ovarian syndrome?**
  Author(s): Cibula D, Hill M, Fanta M, Sindelka G, Zivny J.
  Source: Human Reproduction (Oxford, England). 2001 May; 16(5): 940-4.
  http://www.ncbi.nlm.nih.gov:80/entrez/query.fcgi?cmd=Retrieve&db=PubMed&list_uids=11331641&dopt=Abstract

- **Dysfunction of the growth hormone/insulin-like growth factor-I axis in women with polycystic ovarian syndrome.**
  Author(s): Piaditis GP, Kounadi TG, Rangou DB, Trovas GP, Kaklas NA, Tzonou AJ, Chlouverakis CS.
  Source: Clinical Endocrinology. 1995 June; 42(6): 635-40.
  http://www.ncbi.nlm.nih.gov:80/entrez/query.fcgi?cmd=Retrieve&db=PubMed&list_uids=7634505&dopt=Abstract

- **Dyslipidaemia in polycystic ovarian syndrome: different groups, different aetiologies?**
  Author(s): Meirow D, Raz I, Yossepowitch O, Brzezinski A, Rosler A, Schenker JG, Berry EM.
  Source: Human Reproduction (Oxford, England). 1996 September; 11(9): 1848-53.
  http://www.ncbi.nlm.nih.gov:80/entrez/query.fcgi?cmd=Retrieve&db=PubMed&list_uids=8921052&dopt=Abstract

- **Dysregulation of cytochrome P450c 17 alpha as the cause of polycystic ovarian syndrome.**
  Author(s): Rosenfield RL, Barnes RB, Cara JF, Lucky AW.
  Source: Fertility and Sterility. 1990 May; 53(5): 785-91. Review.
  http://www.ncbi.nlm.nih.gov:80/entrez/query.fcgi?cmd=Retrieve&db=PubMed&list_uids=2185040&dopt=Abstract

- **'Early coasting' in patients with polycystic ovarian syndrome is consistent with good clinical outcome.**
  Author(s): Egbase PE, Al-Sharhan M, Grudzinskas JG.
  Source: Human Reproduction (Oxford, England). 2002 May; 17(5): 1212-6.
  http://www.ncbi.nlm.nih.gov:80/entrez/query.fcgi?cmd=Retrieve&db=PubMed&list_uids=11980740&dopt=Abstract

- **Early metabolic abnormalities in adolescent girls with polycystic ovarian syndrome.**
  Author(s): Lewy VD, Danadian K, Witchel SF, Arslanian S.
  Source: The Journal of Pediatrics. 2001 January; 138(1): 38-44.
  http://www.ncbi.nlm.nih.gov:80/entrez/query.fcgi?cmd=Retrieve&db=PubMed&list_uids=11148510&dopt=Abstract

- **Effect of feeding on growth hormone response to growth hormone-releasing hormone in polycystic ovarian syndrome: relation with body weight and hyperinsulinism.**
    Author(s): Villa P, Soranna L, Mancini A, De Marinis L, Valle D, Mancuso S, Lanzone A.
    Source: Human Reproduction (Oxford, England). 2001 March; 16(3): 430-4.
    http://www.ncbi.nlm.nih.gov:80/entrez/query.fcgi?cmd=Retrieve&db=PubMed&list_uids=11228207&dopt=Abstract

- **Effect of gonadotrophin-releasing hormone agonist treatment on growth hormone secretion in women with polycystic ovarian syndrome.**
    Author(s): Kaltsas T, Pontikides N, Krassas GE, Seferiadis K, Lolis D, Messinis IE.
    Source: Human Reproduction (Oxford, England). 1998 January; 13(1): 22-6.
    http://www.ncbi.nlm.nih.gov:80/entrez/query.fcgi?cmd=Retrieve&db=PubMed&list_uids=9512222&dopt=Abstract

- **Effects of an oral contraceptive containing cyproterone acetate (Diane-35) on the symptoms, hormone profile, and ovarian volume of hirsute women with polycystic ovarian syndrome.**
    Author(s): Prelevic GM, Puzigaca Z, Balint-Peric LA.
    Source: Annals of the New York Academy of Sciences. 1993 May 28; 687: 255-62.
    http://www.ncbi.nlm.nih.gov:80/entrez/query.fcgi?cmd=Retrieve&db=PubMed&list_uids=8323181&dopt=Abstract

- **Effects of metformin therapy on hyperandrogenism in women with polycystic ovarian syndrome.**
    Author(s): Kazerooni T, Dehghan-Kooshkghazi M.
    Source: Gynecological Endocrinology : the Official Journal of the International Society of Gynecological Endocrinology. 2003 February; 17(1): 51-6.
    http://www.ncbi.nlm.nih.gov:80/entrez/query.fcgi?cmd=Retrieve&db=PubMed&list_uids=12724019&dopt=Abstract

- **Efficacy of low dose purified FSH in ovulation induction following pituitary desensitization in polycystic ovarian syndrome.**
    Author(s): Buckler HM, Critchley HO, Cantrill JA, Shalet SM, Anderson DC, Robertson WR.
    Source: Clinical Endocrinology. 1993 February; 38(2): 209-17.
    http://www.ncbi.nlm.nih.gov:80/entrez/query.fcgi?cmd=Retrieve&db=PubMed&list_uids=8435902&dopt=Abstract

- **Efficacy of the combination ethinyl oestradiol and cyproterone acetate on endocrine, clinical and ultrasonographic profile in polycystic ovarian syndrome.**
    Author(s): Falsetti L, Gambera A, Tisi G.
    Source: Human Reproduction (Oxford, England). 2001 January; 16(1): 36-42.
    http://www.ncbi.nlm.nih.gov:80/entrez/query.fcgi?cmd=Retrieve&db=PubMed&list_uids=11139533&dopt=Abstract

- **Elevated endometrial androgen receptor expression in women with polycystic ovarian syndrome.**
  Author(s): Apparao KB, Lovely LP, Gui Y, Lininger RA, Lessey BA.
  Source: Biology of Reproduction. 2002 February; 66(2): 297-304.
  http://www.ncbi.nlm.nih.gov:80/entrez/query.fcgi?cmd=Retrieve&db=PubMed&list_uids=11804942&dopt=Abstract

- **Endocrine changes after laparoscopic ovarian cautery in polycystic ovarian syndrome.**
  Author(s): Greenblatt E, Casper RF.
  Source: American Journal of Obstetrics and Gynecology. 1987 February; 156(2): 279-85.
  http://www.ncbi.nlm.nih.gov:80/entrez/query.fcgi?cmd=Retrieve&db=PubMed&list_uids=2950757&dopt=Abstract

- **Endometrial carcinoma in a young patient with polycystic ovarian syndrome: first suspected at time of embryo transfer.**
  Author(s): Salha O, Martin-Hirsch P, Lane G, Sharma V.
  Source: Human Reproduction (Oxford, England). 1997 May; 12(5): 959-62.
  http://www.ncbi.nlm.nih.gov:80/entrez/query.fcgi?cmd=Retrieve&db=PubMed&list_uids=9194647&dopt=Abstract

- **Evaluation and therapy of polycystic ovarian syndrome.**
  Author(s): Loy R, Seibel MM.
  Source: Endocrinology and Metabolism Clinics of North America. 1988 December; 17(4): 785-813. Review.
  http://www.ncbi.nlm.nih.gov:80/entrez/query.fcgi?cmd=Retrieve&db=PubMed&list_uids=3143568&dopt=Abstract

- **Evaluation of ovarian cysts following GnRH-a treatment in patients with polycystic ovarian syndrome.**
  Author(s): Gregoriou O, Vitoratos N, Konidaris S, Papadias C, Chryssikopoulos A.
  Source: Gynecologic and Obstetric Investigation. 1998; 46(4): 252-5.
  http://www.ncbi.nlm.nih.gov:80/entrez/query.fcgi?cmd=Retrieve&db=PubMed&list_uids=9813444&dopt=Abstract

- **Evidence for a defect in insulin metabolism in hyperandrogenic women with polycystic ovarian syndrome.**
  Author(s): Buffington CK, Kitabchi AE.
  Source: Metabolism: Clinical and Experimental. 1994 November; 43(11): 1367-72.
  http://www.ncbi.nlm.nih.gov:80/entrez/query.fcgi?cmd=Retrieve&db=PubMed&list_uids=7968591&dopt=Abstract

- **Evidence of a distinct derangement of opioid tone in hyperinsulinemic patients with polycystic ovarian syndrome: relationship with insulin and luteinizing hormone secretion.**
  Author(s): Lanzone A, Fulghesu AM, Cucinelli F, Ciampelli M, Caruso A, Mancuso S.
  Source: The Journal of Clinical Endocrinology and Metabolism. 1995 December; 80(12): 3501-6.
  http://www.ncbi.nlm.nih.gov:80/entrez/query.fcgi?cmd=Retrieve&db=PubMed&list_uids=8530590&dopt=Abstract

- **Expression of inhibin alpha, beta A and beta B messenger ribonucleic acids in the normal human ovary and in polycystic ovarian syndrome.**
  Author(s): Jaatinen TA, Penttila TL, Kaipia A, Ekfors T, Parvinen M, Toppari J.
  Source: The Journal of Endocrinology. 1994 October; 143(1): 127-37.
  http://www.ncbi.nlm.nih.gov:80/entrez/query.fcgi?cmd=Retrieve&db=PubMed&list_uids=7964311&dopt=Abstract

- **Expression of inhibin/activin system messenger ribonucleic acids and proteins in ovarian follicles from women with polycystic ovarian syndrome.**
  Author(s): Roberts VJ, Barth S, el-Roeiy A, Yen SS.
  Source: The Journal of Clinical Endocrinology and Metabolism. 1994 November; 79(5): 1434-9.
  http://www.ncbi.nlm.nih.gov:80/entrez/query.fcgi?cmd=Retrieve&db=PubMed&list_uids=7962340&dopt=Abstract

- **Extremely high levels of estradiol and testosterone in a case of polycystic ovarian syndrome. Hormone and clinical similarities with the phenotype of the alpha estrogen receptor null mice.**
  Author(s): Bartolone L, Smedile G, Arcoraci V, Trimarchi F, Benvenga S.
  Source: J Endocrinol Invest. 2000 July-August; 23(7): 467-72.
  http://www.ncbi.nlm.nih.gov:80/entrez/query.fcgi?cmd=Retrieve&db=PubMed&list_uids=11005272&dopt=Abstract

- **Factors affecting the outcome of laparoscopic ovarian drilling for polycystic ovarian syndrome in women with anovulatory infertility.**
  Author(s): Li TC, Saravelos H, Chow MS, Chisabingo R, Cooke ID.
  Source: British Journal of Obstetrics and Gynaecology. 1998 March; 105(3): 338-44.
  http://www.ncbi.nlm.nih.gov:80/entrez/query.fcgi?cmd=Retrieve&db=PubMed&list_uids=9532997&dopt=Abstract

- **Familial clustering in the polycystic ovarian syndrome.**
  Author(s): Lunde O, Magnus P, Sandvik L, Hoglo S.
  Source: Gynecologic and Obstetric Investigation. 1989; 28(1): 23-30.
  http://www.ncbi.nlm.nih.gov:80/entrez/query.fcgi?cmd=Retrieve&db=PubMed&list_uids=2777131&dopt=Abstract

- **Feedback inhibition of insulin secretion and insulin resistance in polycystic ovarian syndrome with and without obesity.**
  Author(s): Sinagra D, Scarpitta AM, Brigandi M, D'Acquisto G.
  Source: Eur Rev Med Pharmacol Sci. 1997 September-October; 1(5): 167-71.
  http://www.ncbi.nlm.nih.gov:80/entrez/query.fcgi?cmd=Retrieve&db=PubMed&list_uids=9630759&dopt=Abstract

- **Follicular development and hormone concentrations following recombinant FSH administration for anovulation associated with polycystic ovarian syndrome: prospective, randomized comparison between low-dose step-up and modified step-down regimens.**
  Author(s): Balasch J, Fabregues F, Creus M, Puerto B, Penarrubia J, Vanrell JA.
  Source: Human Reproduction (Oxford, England). 2001 April; 16(4): 652-6.
  http://www.ncbi.nlm.nih.gov:80/entrez/query.fcgi?cmd=Retrieve&db=PubMed&list_uids=11278212&dopt=Abstract

- **Follicular fluid concentration of leukaemia inhibitory factor is decreased among women with polycystic ovarian syndrome during assisted reproduction cycles.**
  Author(s): Ledee-Bataille N, Lapree-Delage G, Taupin JL, Dubanchet S, Taieb J, Moreau JF, Chaouat G.
  Source: Human Reproduction (Oxford, England). 2001 October; 16(10): 2073-8.
  http://www.ncbi.nlm.nih.gov:80/entrez/query.fcgi?cmd=Retrieve&db=PubMed&list_uids=11574494&dopt=Abstract

- **Galactorrhea and amenorrhea with polycystic ovaries. Del Castillo syndrome or polycystic ovarian syndrome.**
  Author(s): Lavric MV.
  Source: American Journal of Obstetrics and Gynecology. 1969 July 15; 104(6): 814-7.
  http://www.ncbi.nlm.nih.gov:80/entrez/query.fcgi?cmd=Retrieve&db=PubMed&list_uids=5815671&dopt=Abstract

- **GnRH antagonists for treatment of polycystic ovarian syndrome.**
  Author(s): Cardone VS.
  Source: Fertility and Sterility. 2003 July; 80 Suppl 1: S25-31; Discussion S32-4. Review.
  http://www.ncbi.nlm.nih.gov:80/entrez/query.fcgi?cmd=Retrieve&db=PubMed&list_uids=12831915&dopt=Abstract

- **GnRH-agonist therapy in women with the polycystic ovarian syndrome: effects on ovarian volume and on gonadotropin and sex steroid levels.**
  Author(s): Dale PO, Tanbo T, Haug E, Abyholm T.
  Source: Gynecological Endocrinology : the Official Journal of the International Society of Gynecological Endocrinology. 1989 December; 3(4): 309-15.
  http://www.ncbi.nlm.nih.gov:80/entrez/query.fcgi?cmd=Retrieve&db=PubMed&list_uids=2516706&dopt=Abstract

- **Gonadotrophin-releasing hormone analogue as an adjunct to gonadotropin therapy for clomiphene-resistant polycystic ovarian syndrome.**
  Author(s): Hughes E, Collins J, Vandekerckhove P.
  Source: Cochrane Database Syst Rev. 2000; (2): Cd000097. Review.
  http://www.ncbi.nlm.nih.gov:80/entrez/query.fcgi?cmd=Retrieve&db=PubMed&list_uids=10796488&dopt=Abstract

- **Gonadotropin and ovarian steroid production in polycystic ovarian syndrome during suppression with a gonadotropin-releasing hormone agonist.**
  Author(s): Tanbo T, Abyholm T, Magnus O, Henriksen T.
  Source: Gynecologic and Obstetric Investigation. 1989; 28(3): 147-51.
  http://www.ncbi.nlm.nih.gov:80/entrez/query.fcgi?cmd=Retrieve&db=PubMed&list_uids=2509303&dopt=Abstract

- **Gonadotropin-releasing hormone agonist reduces the miscarriage rate for pregnancies achieved in women with polycystic ovarian syndrome.**
  Author(s): Homburg R, Levy T, Berkovitz D, Farchi J, Feldberg D, Ashkenazi J, Ben-Rafael Z.
  Source: Fertility and Sterility. 1993 March; 59(3): 527-31.
  http://www.ncbi.nlm.nih.gov:80/entrez/query.fcgi?cmd=Retrieve&db=PubMed&list_uids=8458452&dopt=Abstract

- **Gonadotropins in polycystic ovarian syndrome.**
  Author(s): Fauser BC, De Jong FH.
  Source: Annals of the New York Academy of Sciences. 1993 May 28; 687: 150-61. Review.
  http://www.ncbi.nlm.nih.gov:80/entrez/query.fcgi?cmd=Retrieve&db=PubMed&list_uids=8323170&dopt=Abstract

- **Growth factors and polycystic ovarian syndrome.**
  Author(s): Giudice LC, Morales AJ, Yen SS.
  Source: Semin Reprod Endocrinol. 1996 August; 14(3): 203-8. Review. No Abstract Available.
  http://www.ncbi.nlm.nih.gov:80/entrez/query.fcgi?cmd=Retrieve&db=PubMed&list_uids=8885051&dopt=Abstract

- **Growth hormone response to L-dopa and pyridostigmine in women with polycystic ovarian syndrome.**
  Author(s): Lee EJ, Lee BS, Lee HC, Park KH, Song CH, Huh KB.
  Source: Fertility and Sterility. 1993 July; 60(1): 53-7.
  http://www.ncbi.nlm.nih.gov:80/entrez/query.fcgi?cmd=Retrieve&db=PubMed&list_uids=8513959&dopt=Abstract

- **Growth hormone response to thyrotrophin releasing hormone in women with polycystic ovarian syndrome.**
  Author(s): Kaltsas T, Pontikides N, Krassas GE, Seferiadis K, Lolis D, Messinis IE.
  Source: Human Reproduction (Oxford, England). 1999 November; 14(11): 2704-8.
  http://www.ncbi.nlm.nih.gov:80/entrez/query.fcgi?cmd=Retrieve&db=PubMed&list_uids=10548605&dopt=Abstract

- **High incidence of embryo transfer cancellations in patients with polycystic ovarian syndrome.**
  Author(s): Kodama H, Fukuda J, Karube H, Matsui T, Shimizu Y, Tanaka T.
  Source: Human Reproduction (Oxford, England). 1995 August; 10(8): 1962-7.
  http://www.ncbi.nlm.nih.gov:80/entrez/query.fcgi?cmd=Retrieve&db=PubMed&list_uids=8567823&dopt=Abstract

- **Hormonal findings in African-American and Caribbean Hispanic girls with premature adrenarche: implications for polycystic ovarian syndrome.**
  Author(s): Banerjee S, Raghavan S, Wasserman EJ, Linder BL, Saenger P, DiMartino-Nardi J.
  Source: Pediatrics. 1998 September; 102(3): E36.
  http://www.ncbi.nlm.nih.gov:80/entrez/query.fcgi?cmd=Retrieve&db=PubMed&list_uids=9724684&dopt=Abstract

- **Hormonal parameters and conception rate during five different types of treatment of polycystic ovarian syndrome.**
  Author(s): Ronnberg L, Ylostalo P, Ruokonen A.
  Source: International Journal of Gynaecology and Obstetrics: the Official Organ of the International Federation of Gynaecology and Obstetrics. 1985 June; 23(3): 177-83.
  http://www.ncbi.nlm.nih.gov:80/entrez/query.fcgi?cmd=Retrieve&db=PubMed&list_uids=2865178&dopt=Abstract

- **Hormonal responses to physical exercise in patients with polycystic ovarian syndrome.**
  Author(s): Jaatinen TA, Anttila L, Erkkola R, Koskinen P, Laippala P, Ruutiainen K, Scheinin M, Irjala K.
  Source: Fertility and Sterility. 1993 August; 60(2): 262-7.
  http://www.ncbi.nlm.nih.gov:80/entrez/query.fcgi?cmd=Retrieve&db=PubMed&list_uids=8339821&dopt=Abstract

- **How common are polycystic ovaries and the polycystic ovarian syndrome in women with Cushing's syndrome?**
  Author(s): Kaltsas GA, Korbonits M, Isidori AM, Webb JA, Trainer PJ, Monson JP, Besser GM, Grossman AB.
  Source: Clinical Endocrinology. 2000 October; 53(4): 493-500.
  http://www.ncbi.nlm.nih.gov:80/entrez/query.fcgi?cmd=Retrieve&db=PubMed&list_uids=11012575&dopt=Abstract

- **How IGF-I and IGF-I binding protein can be modulated in polycystic ovarian syndrome.**
  Author(s): Laatikainen T.
  Source: Annals of the New York Academy of Sciences. 1993 May 28; 687: 90-7. Review.
  http://www.ncbi.nlm.nih.gov:80/entrez/query.fcgi?cmd=Retrieve&db=PubMed&list_uids=7686730&dopt=Abstract

- **Hyperinsulinemia does not influence androgens/estrogens ratio in patients with polycystic ovarian syndrome.**
  Author(s): Panidis DK, Rousso DH, Matalliotakis IM, Kourtis AI, Vlassis GD, Koumantakis EE.
  Source: Int J Fertil Womens Med. 1999 November-December; 44(6): 301-6.
  http://www.ncbi.nlm.nih.gov:80/entrez/query.fcgi?cmd=Retrieve&db=PubMed&list_uids=10617252&dopt=Abstract

- **Hyperinsulinism and insulin resistance in polycystic ovarian syndrome: a verification using oral glucose, I.V. Glucose and tolbutamide.**
  Author(s): Cotrozzi G, Matteini M, Relli P, Lazzari T.
  Source: Acta Diabetol Lat. 1983 April-June; 20(2): 135-42.
  http://www.ncbi.nlm.nih.gov:80/entrez/query.fcgi?cmd=Retrieve&db=PubMed&list_uids=6224386&dopt=Abstract

- **Hypermelatoninemia in women with polycystic ovarian syndrome.**
  Author(s): Tarquini R, Bruni V, Perfetto F, Bigozzi L, Tapparini L, Tarquini B.
  Source: The European Journal of Contraception & Reproductive Health Care : the Official Journal of the European Society of Contraception. 1996 December; 1(4): 349-50.
  http://www.ncbi.nlm.nih.gov:80/entrez/query.fcgi?cmd=Retrieve&db=PubMed&list_uids=9678118&dopt=Abstract

- **Hyperprolactinemia and polycystic ovarian syndrome.**
  Author(s): Tzingounis VA, Aksu MF, Tsoukalos SG.
  Source: Int J Fertil. 1979; 24(4): 276-80.
  http://www.ncbi.nlm.nih.gov:80/entrez/query.fcgi?cmd=Retrieve&db=PubMed&list_uids=45100&dopt=Abstract

- **Immunohistochemical study of steroidogenesis and cell proliferation in polycystic ovarian syndrome.**
  Author(s): Takayama K, Fukaya T, Sasano H, Funayama Y, Suzuki T, Takaya R, Wada Y, Yajima A.
  Source: Human Reproduction (Oxford, England). 1996 July; 11(7): 1387-92.
  http://www.ncbi.nlm.nih.gov:80/entrez/query.fcgi?cmd=Retrieve&db=PubMed&list_uids=8671472&dopt=Abstract

- **In vitro fertilization following laparoscopic ovarian diathermy in patients with polycystic ovarian syndrome.**
  Author(s): Colacurci N, Zullo F, De Franciscis P, Mollo A, De Placido G.
  Source: Acta Obstetricia Et Gynecologica Scandinavica. 1997 July; 76(6): 555-8.
  http://www.ncbi.nlm.nih.gov:80/entrez/query.fcgi?cmd=Retrieve&db=PubMed&list_uids=9246962&dopt=Abstract

- **Incidence and treatment of metabolic syndrome in newly referred women with confirmed polycystic ovarian syndrome.**
  Author(s): Glueck CJ, Papanna R, Wang P, Goldenberg N, Sieve-Smith L.
  Source: Metabolism: Clinical and Experimental. 2003 July; 52(7): 908-15.
  http://www.ncbi.nlm.nih.gov:80/entrez/query.fcgi?cmd=Retrieve&db=PubMed&list_uids=12870169&dopt=Abstract

- **Increased 5alpha-reductase and normal 11beta-hydroxysteroid dehydrogenase metabolism of C19 and C21 steroids in a young population with polycystic ovarian syndrome.**
  Author(s): Chin D, Shackleton C, Prasad VK, Kohn B, David R, Imperato-McGinley J, Cohen H, McMahon DJ, Oberfield SE.
  Source: J Pediatr Endocrinol Metab. 2000 March; 13(3): 253-9.
  http://www.ncbi.nlm.nih.gov:80/entrez/query.fcgi?cmd=Retrieve&db=PubMed&list_uids=10714750&dopt=Abstract

- **Increased number of IGF-I receptors on erythrocytes of women with polycystic ovarian syndrome.**
  Author(s): Gdansky E, Diamant YZ, Laron Z, Silbergeld A, Kaplan B, Eshet R.
  Source: Clinical Endocrinology. 1997 August; 47(2): 185-90.
  http://www.ncbi.nlm.nih.gov:80/entrez/query.fcgi?cmd=Retrieve&db=PubMed&list_uids=9302393&dopt=Abstract

- **Induction of ovulation by pulsatile LH-RH administration in polycystic ovarian syndrome.**
  Author(s): Bolanowski M, Grabinski M, Milewicz A, Zalewski J.
  Source: Endokrynol Pol. 1989; 40(6): 281-4. No Abstract Available.
  http://www.ncbi.nlm.nih.gov:80/entrez/query.fcgi?cmd=Retrieve&db=PubMed&list_uids=2485729&dopt=Abstract

- **Induction of ovulation with gonadotropins in patients with polycystic ovarian syndrome.**
  Author(s): Caruso A, Lanzone A, Fulghesu AM, Guida C, Apa R, Andreani CL, Mancuso S.
  Source: Contrib Gynecol Obstet. 1991; 18: 42-53. No Abstract Available.
  http://www.ncbi.nlm.nih.gov:80/entrez/query.fcgi?cmd=Retrieve&db=PubMed&list_uids=1935128&dopt=Abstract

- **Induction of ovulation with purified urinary follicle-stimulating hormone in patients with polycystic ovarian syndrome.**
  Author(s): Garcea N, Campo S, Panetta V, Venneri M, Siccardi P, Dargenio R, De Tomasi F.
  Source: American Journal of Obstetrics and Gynecology. 1985 March 1; 151(5): 635-40.
  http://www.ncbi.nlm.nih.gov:80/entrez/query.fcgi?cmd=Retrieve&db=PubMed&list_uids=3919586&dopt=Abstract

- **Inhibin A and inhibin B in women with polycystic ovarian syndrome during treatment with FSH to induce mono-ovulation.**
  Author(s): Anderson RA, Groome NP, Baird DT.
  Source: Clinical Endocrinology. 1998 May; 48(5): 577-84.
  http://www.ncbi.nlm.nih.gov:80/entrez/query.fcgi?cmd=Retrieve&db=PubMed&list_uids=9666869&dopt=Abstract

- **Insulin and insulin-like growth factor-I responsiveness in polycystic ovarian syndrome.**
  Author(s): Buyalos RP, Geffner ME, Bersch N, Judd HL, Watanabe RM, Bergman RN, Golde DW.
  Source: Fertility and Sterility. 1992 April; 57(4): 796-803.
  http://www.ncbi.nlm.nih.gov:80/entrez/query.fcgi?cmd=Retrieve&db=PubMed&list_uids=1555690&dopt=Abstract

- **Insulin resistance and polycystic ovarian syndrome.**
  Author(s): Dewailly D, Cortet-Rudelli C.
  Source: Hormone Research. 1992; 38(1-2): 41-5. Review.
  http://www.ncbi.nlm.nih.gov:80/entrez/query.fcgi?cmd=Retrieve&db=PubMed&list_uids=1306514&dopt=Abstract

- **Insulin resistance in polycystic ovarian syndrome.**
  Author(s): Dunaif A.
  Source: Annals of the New York Academy of Sciences. 1993 May 28; 687: 60-4. Review.
  http://www.ncbi.nlm.nih.gov:80/entrez/query.fcgi?cmd=Retrieve&db=PubMed&list_uids=8323191&dopt=Abstract

- **Insulin sensitivity, insulin secretion, and metabolic and hormonal parameters in healthy women and women with polycystic ovarian syndrome.**
  Author(s): Morin-Papunen LC, Vauhkonen I, Koivunen RM, Ruokonen A, Tapanainen JS.
  Source: Human Reproduction (Oxford, England). 2000 June; 15(6): 1266-74.
  http://www.ncbi.nlm.nih.gov:80/entrez/query.fcgi?cmd=Retrieve&db=PubMed&list_uids=10831553&dopt=Abstract

- **Interface between extra- and intraovarian factors in polycystic ovarian syndrome.**
  Author(s): Yen SS, Laughlin GA, Morales AJ.
  Source: Annals of the New York Academy of Sciences. 1993 May 28; 687: 98-111. Review.
  http://www.ncbi.nlm.nih.gov:80/entrez/query.fcgi?cmd=Retrieve&db=PubMed&list_uids=8323193&dopt=Abstract

- **Interrelationship between ultrasonography and biology in the diagnosis of polycystic ovarian syndrome.**
  Author(s): Dewailly D, Duhamel A, Robert Y, Ardaens Y, Beuscart R, Lemaitre L, Fossati P.
  Source: Annals of the New York Academy of Sciences. 1993 May 28; 687: 206-16.
  http://www.ncbi.nlm.nih.gov:80/entrez/query.fcgi?cmd=Retrieve&db=PubMed&list_uids=8323174&dopt=Abstract

- **Investigations on the genetic polymorphism in the region of CYP17 gene encoding 5'-UTR in patients with polycystic ovarian syndrome.**
  Author(s): Marszalek B, Lacinski M, Babych N, Capla E, Biernacka-Lukanty J, Warenik-Szymankiewicz A, Trzeciak WH.
  Source: Gynecological Endocrinology : the Official Journal of the International Society of Gynecological Endocrinology. 2001 April; 15(2): 123-8.
  http://www.ncbi.nlm.nih.gov:80/entrez/query.fcgi?cmd=Retrieve&db=PubMed&list_uids=11379008&dopt=Abstract

- **In-vitro fertilization in infertile women with the polycystic ovarian syndrome.**
  Author(s): Dale PO, Tanbo T, Abyholm T.
  Source: Human Reproduction (Oxford, England). 1991 February; 6(2): 238-41.
  http://www.ncbi.nlm.nih.gov:80/entrez/query.fcgi?cmd=Retrieve&db=PubMed&list_uids=1905314&dopt=Abstract

- **In-vitro progesterone production of human granulosa--luteal cells: the impact of different stimulation protocols, poor ovarian response and polycystic ovarian syndrome.**
  Author(s): Hamori M, Torok A, Zwirner M, Batteux C, Schinkmann W, Bodis J.
  Source: Human Reproduction (Oxford, England). 1992 May; 7(5): 592-6.
  http://www.ncbi.nlm.nih.gov:80/entrez/query.fcgi?cmd=Retrieve&db=PubMed&list_uids=1639973&dopt=Abstract

- **In-vivo ovarian androgen responses to recombinant FSH with and without recombinant LH in polycystic ovarian syndrome.**
  Author(s): Cheung AP, Pride SM, Yuen BH, Sy L.
  Source: Human Reproduction (Oxford, England). 2002 October; 17(10): 2540-7.
  http://www.ncbi.nlm.nih.gov:80/entrez/query.fcgi?cmd=Retrieve&db=PubMed&list_uids=12351525&dopt=Abstract

- **Laparoscopic ovarian diathermy in women with polycystic ovarian syndrome: a retrospective study on the influence of the amount of energy used on the outcome.**
  Author(s): Amer SA, Li TC, Cooke ID.
  Source: Human Reproduction (Oxford, England). 2002 April; 17(4): 1046-51.
  http://www.ncbi.nlm.nih.gov:80/entrez/query.fcgi?cmd=Retrieve&db=PubMed&list_uids=11925403&dopt=Abstract

- **Laparoscopic ovarian drilling in women with polycystic ovarian syndrome.**
  Author(s): Greenblatt EM, Casper RF.
  Source: Prog Clin Biol Res. 1993; 381: 129-38. Review. No Abstract Available.
  http://www.ncbi.nlm.nih.gov:80/entrez/query.fcgi?cmd=Retrieve&db=PubMed&list_uids=8316557&dopt=Abstract

- **Laparoscopic ovarian treatment in infertile patients with polycystic ovarian syndrome (PCOS): endocrine changes and clinical outcome.**
  Author(s): Liguori G, Tolino A, Moccia G, Scognamiglio G, Nappi C.
  Source: Gynecological Endocrinology : the Official Journal of the International Society of Gynecological Endocrinology. 1996 August; 10(4): 257-64.
  http://www.ncbi.nlm.nih.gov:80/entrez/query.fcgi?cmd=Retrieve&db=PubMed&list_uids=8908526&dopt=Abstract

- **Laparoscopic procedures for treatment of infertility related to polycystic ovarian syndrome.**
  Author(s): Cohen J.
  Source: Human Reproduction Update. 1996 July-August; 2(4): 337-44. Review.
  http://www.ncbi.nlm.nih.gov:80/entrez/query.fcgi?cmd=Retrieve&db=PubMed&list_uids=9080230&dopt=Abstract

- **Laparoscopic treatment of polycystic ovarian syndrome.**
  Author(s): Keckstein J.
  Source: Baillieres Clin Obstet Gynaecol. 1989 September; 3(3): 563-81. Review.
  http://www.ncbi.nlm.nih.gov:80/entrez/query.fcgi?cmd=Retrieve&db=PubMed&list_uids=2533011&dopt=Abstract

- **LH levels in women with polycystic ovarian syndrome: have modern assays made them irrelevant?**
  Author(s): Milsom SR, Sowter MC, Carter MA, Knox BS, Gunn AJ.
  Source: Bjog : an International Journal of Obstetrics and Gynaecology. 2003 August; 110(8): 760-4.
  http://www.ncbi.nlm.nih.gov:80/entrez/query.fcgi?cmd=Retrieve&db=PubMed&list_uids=12892688&dopt=Abstract

- **Limited ovarian stimulation (LOS), prevents the recurrence of severe forms of ovarian hyperstimulation syndrome in polycystic ovarian disease.**
  Author(s): El-Sheikh MM, Hussein M, Fouad S, El-Sheikh R, Bauer O, Al-Hasani S.
  Source: European Journal of Obstetrics, Gynecology, and Reproductive Biology. 2001 February; 94(2): 245-9.
  http://www.ncbi.nlm.nih.gov:80/entrez/query.fcgi?cmd=Retrieve&db=PubMed&list_uids=11165733&dopt=Abstract

- **Long term follow-up of patients with polycystic ovarian syndrome after laparoscopic ovarian drilling: clinical outcome.**
  Author(s): Amer SA, Gopalan V, Li TC, Ledger WL, Cooke ID.
  Source: Human Reproduction (Oxford, England). 2002 August; 17(8): 2035-42.
  http://www.ncbi.nlm.nih.gov:80/entrez/query.fcgi?cmd=Retrieve&db=PubMed&list_uids=12151433&dopt=Abstract

- **Long-term clinical effects of ovarian wedge resection in polycystic ovarian syndrome.**
  Author(s): Hjortrup A, Kehlet H, Lockwood K, Hasner E.
  Source: Acta Obstetricia Et Gynecologica Scandinavica. 1983; 62(1): 55-7.
  http://www.ncbi.nlm.nih.gov:80/entrez/query.fcgi?cmd=Retrieve&db=PubMed&list_uids=6858626&dopt=Abstract

- **Long-term follow-up in 206 infertility patients with polycystic ovarian syndrome after laparoscopic electrocautery of the ovarian surface.**
  Author(s): Naether OG, Baukloh V, Fischer R, Kowalczyk T.
  Source: Human Reproduction (Oxford, England). 1994 December; 9(12): 2342-9.
  http://www.ncbi.nlm.nih.gov:80/entrez/query.fcgi?cmd=Retrieve&db=PubMed&list_uids=7714155&dopt=Abstract

- **Long-term GnRH analogue treatment is equivalent to laparoscopic laser diathermy in polycystic ovarian syndrome patients with severe ovarian dysfunction.**
  Author(s): Muenstermann U, Kleinstein J.
  Source: Human Reproduction (Oxford, England). 2000 December; 15(12): 2526-30.
  http://www.ncbi.nlm.nih.gov:80/entrez/query.fcgi?cmd=Retrieve&db=PubMed&list_uids=11098021&dopt=Abstract

- **Long-term naltrexone treatment normalizes the pituitary response to gonadotropin-releasing hormone in polycystic ovarian syndrome.**
  Author(s): Lanzone A, Apa R, Fulghesu AM, Cutillo G, Caruso A, Mancuso S.
  Source: Fertility and Sterility. 1993 April; 59(4): 734-7.
  http://www.ncbi.nlm.nih.gov:80/entrez/query.fcgi?cmd=Retrieve&db=PubMed&list_uids=8458488&dopt=Abstract

- **Low grade chronic inflammation in women with polycystic ovarian syndrome.**
  Author(s): Kelly CC, Lyall H, Petrie JR, Gould GW, Connell JM, Sattar N.
  Source: The Journal of Clinical Endocrinology and Metabolism. 2001 June; 86(6): 2453-5.
  http://www.ncbi.nlm.nih.gov:80/entrez/query.fcgi?cmd=Retrieve&db=PubMed&list_uids=11397838&dopt=Abstract

- **Low-dose gonadotropin therapy in polycystic ovarian syndrome.**
  Author(s): Franks S, Hamilton-Fairley D, Sagle M, Polson D, Kiddy D, Watson H, White D.
  Source: Annals of the New York Academy of Sciences. 1993 May 28; 687: 301-4. Review.
  http://www.ncbi.nlm.nih.gov:80/entrez/query.fcgi?cmd=Retrieve&db=PubMed&list_uids=8323187&dopt=Abstract

- **Maternal serum androgens in pregnant women with polycystic ovarian syndrome: possible implications in prenatal androgenization.**
  Author(s): Sir-Petermann T, Maliqueo M, Angel B, Lara HE, Perez-Bravo F, Recabarren SE.
  Source: Human Reproduction (Oxford, England). 2002 October; 17(10): 2573-9.
  http://www.ncbi.nlm.nih.gov:80/entrez/query.fcgi?cmd=Retrieve&db=PubMed&list_uids=12351531&dopt=Abstract

- **Mechanisms behind lipolytic catecholamine resistance of subcutaneous fat cells in the polycystic ovarian syndrome.**
  Author(s): Faulds G, Ryden M, Ek I, Wahrenberg H, Arner P.
  Source: The Journal of Clinical Endocrinology and Metabolism. 2003 May; 88(5): 2269-73.
  http://www.ncbi.nlm.nih.gov:80/entrez/query.fcgi?cmd=Retrieve&db=PubMed&list_uids=12727985&dopt=Abstract

- **Mechanisms of hypothalamic-pituitary-gonadal disruption in polycystic ovarian syndrome.**
  Author(s): Barontini M, Garcia-Rudaz MC, Veldhuis JD.
  Source: Archives of Medical Research. 2001 November-December; 32(6): 544-52. Review.
  http://www.ncbi.nlm.nih.gov:80/entrez/query.fcgi?cmd=Retrieve&db=PubMed&list_uids=11750729&dopt=Abstract

- **Metformin and FSH for induction of ovulation in women with polycystic ovarian syndrome.**
  Author(s): De Leo V, La Marca A.
  Source: Human Reproduction (Oxford, England). 2002 September; 17(9): 2481-2.
  http://www.ncbi.nlm.nih.gov:80/entrez/query.fcgi?cmd=Retrieve&db=PubMed&list_uids=12202445&dopt=Abstract

- **Mid-follicular phase pulses of inhibin B are absent in polycystic ovarian syndrome and are initiated by successful laparoscopic ovarian diathermy: a possible mechanism regulating emergence of the dominant follicle.**
  Author(s): Lockwood GM, Muttukrishna S, Groome NP, Matthews DR, Ledger WL.
  Source: The Journal of Clinical Endocrinology and Metabolism. 1998 May; 83(5): 1730-5.
  http://www.ncbi.nlm.nih.gov:80/entrez/query.fcgi?cmd=Retrieve&db=PubMed&list_uids=9589683&dopt=Abstract

- **Molecular scanning of the insulin receptor gene in women with polycystic ovarian syndrome.**
  Author(s): Talbot JA, Bicknell EJ, Rajkhowa M, Krook A, O'Rahilly S, Clayton RN.
  Source: The Journal of Clinical Endocrinology and Metabolism. 1996 May; 81(5): 1979-83.
  http://www.ncbi.nlm.nih.gov:80/entrez/query.fcgi?cmd=Retrieve&db=PubMed&list_uids=8626868&dopt=Abstract

- **Myths and facts about polycystic ovarian syndrome.**
  Author(s): Munson BL.
  Source: Nursing. 2002 November; 32(11 Pt 1): 78.
  http://www.ncbi.nlm.nih.gov:80/entrez/query.fcgi?cmd=Retrieve&db=PubMed&list_uids=12518752&dopt=Abstract

- **New approaches to insulin resistance in polycystic ovarian syndrome.**
  Author(s): Davison RM.
  Source: Current Opinion in Obstetrics & Gynecology. 1998 June; 10(3): 193-8. Review.
  http://www.ncbi.nlm.nih.gov:80/entrez/query.fcgi?cmd=Retrieve&db=PubMed&list_uids=9619341&dopt=Abstract

- **New approaches to the study of the neuroendocrine abnormalities of women with the polycystic ovarian syndrome.**
  Author(s): Hall JE, Taylor AE, Martin KA, Crowley WF Jr.
  Source: Annals of the New York Academy of Sciences. 1993 May 28; 687: 182-92. Review.
  http://www.ncbi.nlm.nih.gov:80/entrez/query.fcgi?cmd=Retrieve&db=PubMed&list_uids=8323172&dopt=Abstract

- **New approaches with the FSH threshold principle in polycystic ovarian syndrome.**
  Author(s): Schoemaker J, van Weissenbruch MM, van der Meer M.
  Source: Annals of the New York Academy of Sciences. 1993 May 28; 687: 296-300. Review.
  http://www.ncbi.nlm.nih.gov:80/entrez/query.fcgi?cmd=Retrieve&db=PubMed&list_uids=8323186&dopt=Abstract

- **Nitrendipine treatment in women with polycystic ovarian syndrome: evidence for a lack of effects of calcium channel blockers on insulin, androgens, and sex hormone-binding globulin.**
  Author(s): Pasquali R, Cantobelli S, Vicennati V, Casimirri F, Spinucci G, de Iasio R, Mesini P, Boschi S, Nestler JE.
  Source: The Journal of Clinical Endocrinology and Metabolism. 1995 November; 80(11): 3346-50.
  http://www.ncbi.nlm.nih.gov:80/entrez/query.fcgi?cmd=Retrieve&db=PubMed&list_uids=7593449&dopt=Abstract

- **Nonclassical congenital adrenal hyperplasia and the polycystic ovarian syndrome.**
  Author(s): New MI.
  Source: Annals of the New York Academy of Sciences. 1993 May 28; 687: 193-205.
  http://www.ncbi.nlm.nih.gov:80/entrez/query.fcgi?cmd=Retrieve&db=PubMed&list_uids=8323173&dopt=Abstract

- **Obstetric outcome in women with polycystic ovarian syndrome.**
  Author(s): Kashyap S, Claman P.
  Source: Human Reproduction (Oxford, England). 2001 July; 16(7): 1537.
  http://www.ncbi.nlm.nih.gov:80/entrez/query.fcgi?cmd=Retrieve&db=PubMed&list_uids=11425843&dopt=Abstract

- **Obstetric outcome in women with polycystic ovarian syndrome.**
  Author(s): Mikola M, Hiilesmaa V, Halttunen M, Suhonen L, Tiitinen A.
  Source: Human Reproduction (Oxford, England). 2001 February; 16(2): 226-9.
  http://www.ncbi.nlm.nih.gov:80/entrez/query.fcgi?cmd=Retrieve&db=PubMed&list_uids=11157811&dopt=Abstract

- **Oligodontia of the permanent dentition in two sisters with polycystic ovarian syndrome: case reports.**
  Author(s): Hattab FN, Angmar-Mansson B.
  Source: Oral Surgery, Oral Medicine, Oral Pathology, Oral Radiology, and Endodontics. 1997 October; 84(4): 368-71.
  http://www.ncbi.nlm.nih.gov:80/entrez/query.fcgi?cmd=Retrieve&db=PubMed&list_uids=9347500&dopt=Abstract

- **Oocyte quality and treatment outcome in intracytoplasmic sperm injection cycles of polycystic ovarian syndrome patients.**
  Author(s): Ludwig M, Finas DF, al-Hasani S, Diedrich K, Ortmann O.
  Source: Human Reproduction (Oxford, England). 1999 February; 14(2): 354-8.
  http://www.ncbi.nlm.nih.gov:80/entrez/query.fcgi?cmd=Retrieve&db=PubMed&list_uids=10099978&dopt=Abstract

- **Ovarian hyperstimulation syndrome caused by GnRH-analogue treatment without gonadotropin therapy in a patient with polycystic ovarian syndrome.**
  Author(s): Jirecek S, Nagele F, Huber JC, Wenzl R.
  Source: Acta Obstetricia Et Gynecologica Scandinavica. 1998 October; 77(9): 940-1.
  http://www.ncbi.nlm.nih.gov:80/entrez/query.fcgi?cmd=Retrieve&db=PubMed&list_uids=9808388&dopt=Abstract

- **Ovarian morphology in long-term androgen-treated female to male transsexuals. A human model for the study of polycystic ovarian syndrome?**
  Author(s): Pache TD, Chadha S, Gooren LJ, Hop WC, Jaarsma KW, Dommerholt HB, Fauser BC.
  Source: Histopathology. 1991 November; 19(5): 445-52.
  http://www.ncbi.nlm.nih.gov:80/entrez/query.fcgi?cmd=Retrieve&db=PubMed&list_uids=1757084&dopt=Abstract

- **Ovarian sensitivity to follicle-stimulating hormone during the follicular phase of the human menstrual cycle and in patients with polycystic ovarian syndrome.**
  Author(s): Caruso A, Fortini A, Fulghesu AM, Pistilli E, Cucinelli F, Lanzone A, Mancuso S.
  Source: Fertility and Sterility. 1993 January; 59(1): 115-20.
  http://www.ncbi.nlm.nih.gov:80/entrez/query.fcgi?cmd=Retrieve&db=PubMed&list_uids=8419197&dopt=Abstract

- **Ovarian stimulation with low-dose pure follicle-stimulating hormone in polycystic ovarian syndrome anovulatory patients: effect of long-term pretreatment with gonadotrophin-releasing hormone analogue.**
    Author(s): Vegetti W, Testa G, Ragni G, Parazzini F, Crosignani PG.
    Source: Gynecologic and Obstetric Investigation. 1998; 45(3): 186-9.
    http://www.ncbi.nlm.nih.gov:80/entrez/query.fcgi?cmd=Retrieve&db=PubMed&list_uids=9565144&dopt=Abstract

- **Ovarian wedge resection by minilaparatomy in infertile patients with polycystic ovarian syndrome: a new technique.**
    Author(s): Yildirim M, Noyan V, Bulent Tiras M, Yildiz A, Guner H.
    Source: European Journal of Obstetrics, Gynecology, and Reproductive Biology. 2003 March 26; 107(1): 85-7.
    http://www.ncbi.nlm.nih.gov:80/entrez/query.fcgi?cmd=Retrieve&db=PubMed&list_uids=12593902&dopt=Abstract

- **Ovulation induction by step-down administration of purified urinary follicle-stimulating hormone in patients with polycystic ovarian syndrome.**
    Author(s): Mizunuma H, Takagi T, Yamada K, Andoh K, Ibuki Y, Igarashi M.
    Source: Fertility and Sterility. 1991 June; 55(6): 1195-6.
    http://www.ncbi.nlm.nih.gov:80/entrez/query.fcgi?cmd=Retrieve&db=PubMed&list_uids=1903734&dopt=Abstract

- **Ovulation induction with pulsatile gonadotropin-releasing hormone administration in patients with polycystic ovarian syndrome.**
    Author(s): Ory SJ, London SN, Tyrey L, Hammond CB.
    Source: Fertility and Sterility. 1985 January; 43(1): 20-5.
    http://www.ncbi.nlm.nih.gov:80/entrez/query.fcgi?cmd=Retrieve&db=PubMed&list_uids=3880710&dopt=Abstract

- **Pituitary and adrenal response to ovine corticotropin-releasing hormone in women with polycystic ovarian syndrome.**
    Author(s): Mongioi A, Macchi M, Vicari E, Fornito MC, Calogero AE, Riccioli C, Minacapilli G, Moncada ML, D'Agata R.
    Source: J Endocrinol Invest. 1988 October; 11(9): 637-40.
    http://www.ncbi.nlm.nih.gov:80/entrez/query.fcgi?cmd=Retrieve&db=PubMed&list_uids=3265424&dopt=Abstract

- **Pituitary response to bolus and continuous intravenous infusion of luteinizing hormone-releasing factor in normal women and women with polycystic ovarian syndrome.**
    Author(s): Mortimer RH, Lev-Gur M, Freeman R, Fleischer N.
    Source: American Journal of Obstetrics and Gynecology. 1978 March 15; 130(6): 630-4.
    http://www.ncbi.nlm.nih.gov:80/entrez/query.fcgi?cmd=Retrieve&db=PubMed&list_uids=345810&dopt=Abstract

- **Polycystic kidney disease associated with polycystic ovarian syndrome.**
  Author(s): Segasothy M, Norazlina MY, Ong PH, Jamil M.
  Source: Nephron. 1992; 62(4): 482-3.
  http://www.ncbi.nlm.nih.gov:80/entrez/query.fcgi?cmd=Retrieve&db=PubMed&list_uids=1300452&dopt=Abstract

- **Polycystic ovarian syndrome (PCOS) and insulin resistance.**
  Author(s): Park KH, Kim JY, Ahn CW, Song YD, Lim SK, Lee HC.
  Source: International Journal of Gynaecology and Obstetrics: the Official Organ of the International Federation of Gynaecology and Obstetrics. 2001 September; 74(3): 261-7.
  http://www.ncbi.nlm.nih.gov:80/entrez/query.fcgi?cmd=Retrieve&db=PubMed&list_uids=11543750&dopt=Abstract

- **Polycystic ovarian syndrome and insulin resistance in white and Mexican American women.**
  Author(s): Gokcel A, Bagis T, Zeyneloglu HB.
  Source: American Journal of Obstetrics and Gynecology. 2003 June; 188(6): 1661; Author Reply 1661-2.
  http://www.ncbi.nlm.nih.gov:80/entrez/query.fcgi?cmd=Retrieve&db=PubMed&list_uids=12825010&dopt=Abstract

- **Polycystic ovarian syndrome and insulin resistance in white and Mexican American women: a comparison of two distinct populations.**
  Author(s): Kauffman RP, Baker VM, Dimarino P, Gimpel T, Castracane VD.
  Source: American Journal of Obstetrics and Gynecology. 2002 November; 187(5): 1362-9.
  http://www.ncbi.nlm.nih.gov:80/entrez/query.fcgi?cmd=Retrieve&db=PubMed&list_uids=12439532&dopt=Abstract

- **Polycystic ovarian syndrome and pregnancy.**
  Author(s): Paternoster D, Vanin M.
  Source: Minerva Ginecol. 1997 June; 49(6): 293-7.
  http://www.ncbi.nlm.nih.gov:80/entrez/query.fcgi?cmd=Retrieve&db=PubMed&list_uids=9269124&dopt=Abstract

- **Polycystic ovarian syndrome and the risk of spontaneous abortion following assisted reproductive technology treatment.**
  Author(s): Wang JX, Davies MJ, Norman RJ.
  Source: Human Reproduction (Oxford, England). 2001 December; 16(12): 2606-9.
  http://www.ncbi.nlm.nih.gov:80/entrez/query.fcgi?cmd=Retrieve&db=PubMed&list_uids=11726582&dopt=Abstract

- **Polycystic ovarian syndrome and thrombophilia.**
  Author(s): Tsanadis G, Vartholomatos G, Korkontzelos I, Avgoustatos F, Kakosimos G, Sotiriadis A, Tatsioni A, Eleftheriou A, Lolis D.
  Source: Human Reproduction (Oxford, England). 2002 February; 17(2): 314-9.
  http://www.ncbi.nlm.nih.gov:80/entrez/query.fcgi?cmd=Retrieve&db=PubMed&list_uids=11821270&dopt=Abstract

- **Polycystic ovarian syndrome in identical twins.**
  Author(s): Hutton C, Clark F.
  Source: Postgraduate Medical Journal. 1984 January; 60(699): 64-5.
  http://www.ncbi.nlm.nih.gov:80/entrez/query.fcgi?cmd=Retrieve&db=PubMed&list_uids=6538041&dopt=Abstract

- **Polycystic ovarian syndrome in women with epilepsy: a review.**
  Author(s): Duncan S.
  Source: Epilepsia. 2001; 42 Suppl 3: 60-5. Review.
  http://www.ncbi.nlm.nih.gov:80/entrez/query.fcgi?cmd=Retrieve&db=PubMed&list_uids=11520327&dopt=Abstract

- **Polycystic ovarian syndrome in women with epilepsy: epileptic or iatrogenic?**
  Author(s): Herzog AG.
  Source: Annals of Neurology. 1996 May; 39(5): 559-60.
  http://www.ncbi.nlm.nih.gov:80/entrez/query.fcgi?cmd=Retrieve&db=PubMed&list_uids=8619539&dopt=Abstract

- **Polycystic ovarian syndrome treated by laser through the laparoscope.**
  Author(s): Huber J, Hosmann J, Spona J.
  Source: Lancet. 1988 July 23; 2(8604): 215.
  http://www.ncbi.nlm.nih.gov:80/entrez/query.fcgi?cmd=Retrieve&db=PubMed&list_uids=2899681&dopt=Abstract

- **Polycystic ovarian syndrome treated by ovarian electrocautery through the laparoscope.**
  Author(s): Gjonnaess H.
  Source: Fertility and Sterility. 1984 January; 41(1): 20-5.
  http://www.ncbi.nlm.nih.gov:80/entrez/query.fcgi?cmd=Retrieve&db=PubMed&list_uids=6692959&dopt=Abstract

- **Polycystic ovarian syndrome with unilateral cystic teratoma.**
  Author(s): Cooke CW, McEvoy D, Wallach EE.
  Source: Obstetrics and Gynecology. 1972 May; 39(5): 789-94.
  http://www.ncbi.nlm.nih.gov:80/entrez/query.fcgi?cmd=Retrieve&db=PubMed&list_uids=4336822&dopt=Abstract

- **Polycystic ovarian syndrome. A challenge for occupational health nursing.**
  Author(s): Kelley LS.
  Source: Aaohn Journal : Official Journal of the American Association of Occupational Health Nurses. 2003 January; 51(1): 23-7. Review.
  http://www.ncbi.nlm.nih.gov:80/entrez/query.fcgi?cmd=Retrieve&db=PubMed&list_uids=12596342&dopt=Abstract

- **Polycystic ovarian syndrome. Evidence for an autoimmune mechanism in some cases.**
  Author(s): van Gelderen CJ, Gomes dos Santos ML.
  Source: J Reprod Med. 1993 May; 38(5): 381-6.
  http://www.ncbi.nlm.nih.gov:80/entrez/query.fcgi?cmd=Retrieve&db=PubMed&list_uids=8320676&dopt=Abstract

- **Polycystic ovarian syndrome. Preventing long-term health effects.**
  Author(s): Carcio H.
  Source: Adv Nurse Pract. 2000 November; 8(11): 38-43; Quiz 43-5. Review.
  http://www.ncbi.nlm.nih.gov:80/entrez/query.fcgi?cmd=Retrieve&db=PubMed&list_uids=12397915&dopt=Abstract

- **Polycystic ovarian syndrome: a follow-up study on fertility and menstrual pattern in 149 patients 15-25 years after ovarian wedge resection.**
  Author(s): Lunde O, Djoseland O, Grottum P.
  Source: Human Reproduction (Oxford, England). 2001 July; 16(7): 1479-85.
  http://www.ncbi.nlm.nih.gov:80/entrez/query.fcgi?cmd=Retrieve&db=PubMed&list_uids=11425833&dopt=Abstract

- **Polycystic ovarian syndrome: a new perspective.**
  Author(s): Ahmed Y, Akhtar AS, Qureshi F, Qureshi F, Anjum Q, Anhalt H.
  Source: J Pak Med Assoc. 2003 February; 53(2): 72-7. Review. No Abstract Available.
  http://www.ncbi.nlm.nih.gov:80/entrez/query.fcgi?cmd=Retrieve&db=PubMed&list_uids=12705489&dopt=Abstract

- **Polycystic ovarian syndrome: assessment with color Doppler angiography and three-dimensional ultrasonography.**
  Author(s): Dolz M, Osborne NG, Blanes J, Raga F, Abad-Velasco L, Villalobos A, Pellicer A, Bonilla-Musoles F.
  Source: Journal of Ultrasound in Medicine : Official Journal of the American Institute of Ultrasound in Medicine. 1999 April; 18(4): 303-13.
  http://www.ncbi.nlm.nih.gov:80/entrez/query.fcgi?cmd=Retrieve&db=PubMed&list_uids=10206219&dopt=Abstract

- **Polycystic ovarian syndrome: evidence that flutamide restores sensitivity of the gonadotropin-releasing hormone pulse generator to inhibition by estradiol and progesterone.**
  Author(s): Eagleson CA, Gingrich MB, Pastor CL, Arora TK, Burt CM, Evans WS, Marshall JC.
  Source: The Journal of Clinical Endocrinology and Metabolism. 2000 November; 85(11): 4047-52.
  http://www.ncbi.nlm.nih.gov:80/entrez/query.fcgi?cmd=Retrieve&db=PubMed&list_uids=11095431&dopt=Abstract

- **Polycystic ovarian syndrome: is community care appropriate?**
  Author(s): Gupta S.
  Source: Int J Clin Pract. 1999 July-August; 53(5): 359-62. Review.
  http://www.ncbi.nlm.nih.gov:80/entrez/query.fcgi?cmd=Retrieve&db=PubMed&list_uids=10695100&dopt=Abstract

- **Polycystic ovarian syndrome: pregnancy outcome following in vitro fertilization-embryo transfer.**
  Author(s): Alcalay M, Bider D, Lipitz S, Mashiach S, Levran D, Dor J.
  Source: Gynecological Endocrinology : the Official Journal of the International Society of Gynecological Endocrinology. 1995 June; 9(2): 119-23.
  http://www.ncbi.nlm.nih.gov:80/entrez/query.fcgi?cmd=Retrieve&db=PubMed&list_uids=7502687&dopt=Abstract

- **Polycystic ovarian syndrome: safety and effectiveness of stepwise and low-dose administration of purified follicle-stimulating hormone.**
  Author(s): Shoham Z, Patel A, Jacobs HS.
  Source: Fertility and Sterility. 1991 June; 55(6): 1051-6.
  http://www.ncbi.nlm.nih.gov:80/entrez/query.fcgi?cmd=Retrieve&db=PubMed&list_uids=1903725&dopt=Abstract

- **Polycystic ovarian syndrome: the metabolic syndrome comes to gynaecology.**
  Author(s): Hopkinson ZE, Sattar N, Fleming R, Greer IA.
  Source: Bmj (Clinical Research Ed.). 1998 August 1; 317(7154): 329-32. Review.
  http://www.ncbi.nlm.nih.gov:80/entrez/query.fcgi?cmd=Retrieve&db=PubMed&list_uids=9685283&dopt=Abstract

- **Polycystic ovarian syndrome; a retrospective study of the therapeutic effect of ovarian wedge resection after unsuccessful treatment with clomiphene citrate.**
  Author(s): Lunde O.
  Source: Ann Chir Gynaecol. 1982; 71(6): 330-3.
  http://www.ncbi.nlm.nih.gov:80/entrez/query.fcgi?cmd=Retrieve&db=PubMed&list_uids=7159002&dopt=Abstract

- **Polycystic ovarian syndrome--an update on diagnostic evaluation.**
  Author(s): Carmina E.
  Source: J Indian Med Assoc. 1999 February; 97(2): 41-2. No Abstract Available.
  http://www.ncbi.nlm.nih.gov:80/entrez/query.fcgi?cmd=Retrieve&db=PubMed&list_uids=10549191&dopt=Abstract

- **Polycystic ovarian syndrome--relationship to epilepsy and antiepileptic drug therapy.**
  Author(s): Joffe H, Taylor AE, Hall JE.
  Source: The Journal of Clinical Endocrinology and Metabolism. 2001 July; 86(7): 2946-9. Review.
  http://www.ncbi.nlm.nih.gov:80/entrez/query.fcgi?cmd=Retrieve&db=PubMed&list_uids=11443148&dopt=Abstract

- **Polycystic ovaries in patients with hypogonadotropic hypogonadism: similarity of ovarian response to gonadotropin stimulation in patients with polycystic ovarian syndrome.**
  Author(s): Shoham Z, Conway GS, Patel A, Jacobs HS.
  Source: Fertility and Sterility. 1992 July; 58(1): 37-45.
  http://www.ncbi.nlm.nih.gov:80/entrez/query.fcgi?cmd=Retrieve&db=PubMed&list_uids=1624021&dopt=Abstract

- **Post-operative adhesions after laparoscopic electrosurgical treatment for polycystic ovarian syndrome with the application of Interceed to one ovary: a prospective randomized controlled study.**
  Author(s): Saravelos H, Li TC.
  Source: Human Reproduction (Oxford, England). 1996 May; 11(5): 992-7.
  http://www.ncbi.nlm.nih.gov:80/entrez/query.fcgi?cmd=Retrieve&db=PubMed&list_uids=8671376&dopt=Abstract

- **Predictive value of serum and follicular fluid leptin concentrations during assisted reproductive cycles in normal women and in women with the polycystic ovarian syndrome.**
  Author(s): Mantzoros CS, Cramer DW, Liberman RF, Barbieri RL.
  Source: Human Reproduction (Oxford, England). 2000 March; 15(3): 539-44.
  http://www.ncbi.nlm.nih.gov:80/entrez/query.fcgi?cmd=Retrieve&db=PubMed&list_uids=10686193&dopt=Abstract

- **Pregnancy after transfer of cryopreserved embryos in clomiphene citrate resistant polycystic ovarian syndrome.**
  Author(s): Dale PO, Tanbo T, Kjekshus E, Abyholm T.
  Source: Fertility and Sterility. 1990 February; 53(2): 362-4.
  http://www.ncbi.nlm.nih.gov:80/entrez/query.fcgi?cmd=Retrieve&db=PubMed&list_uids=2153591&dopt=Abstract

- **Pregnancy and delivery after cryopreservation of zygotes produced by in-vitro matured oocytes retrieved from a woman with polycystic ovarian syndrome.**
  Author(s): Chian RC, Gulekli B, Buckett WM, Tan SL.
  Source: Human Reproduction (Oxford, England). 2001 August; 16(8): 1700-2.
  http://www.ncbi.nlm.nih.gov:80/entrez/query.fcgi?cmd=Retrieve&db=PubMed&list_uids=11473967&dopt=Abstract

- **Prevalence of and etiological factors in polycystic ovarian syndrome.**
  Author(s): Franks S, White DM.
  Source: Annals of the New York Academy of Sciences. 1993 May 28; 687: 112-4. Review.
  http://www.ncbi.nlm.nih.gov:80/entrez/query.fcgi?cmd=Retrieve&db=PubMed&list_uids=8323165&dopt=Abstract

- **Prevalence of gestational diabetes mellitus in polycystic ovarian syndrome (PCOS) patients pregnant after ovulation induction with gonadotrophins.**
  Author(s): Vollenhoven B, Clark S, Kovacs G, Burger H, Healy D.
  Source: The Australian & New Zealand Journal of Obstetrics & Gynaecology. 2000 February; 40(1): 54-8.
  http://www.ncbi.nlm.nih.gov:80/entrez/query.fcgi?cmd=Retrieve&db=PubMed&list_uids=10870780&dopt=Abstract

- **Primary amenorrhoea associated with polycystic ovarian syndrome.**
  Author(s): Valkov IM, Dokumov SI.
  Source: Reproduccion. 1981 April-June; 5(2): 119-26.
  http://www.ncbi.nlm.nih.gov:80/entrez/query.fcgi?cmd=Retrieve&db=PubMed&list_uids=6790313&dopt=Abstract

- **Prolactin release in polycystic ovarian syndrome.**
  Author(s): Minakami H, Abe N, Oka N, Kimura K, Tamura T, Tamada T.
  Source: Endocrinol Jpn. 1988 April; 35(2): 303-10.
  http://www.ncbi.nlm.nih.gov:80/entrez/query.fcgi?cmd=Retrieve&db=PubMed&list_uids=3145187&dopt=Abstract

- **Prolonged opioid blockade with naltrexone and luteinizing hormone modifications in women with polycystic ovarian syndrome.**
  Author(s): Cagnacci A, Soldani R, Paoletti AM, Falqui A, Melis GB.
  Source: Fertility and Sterility. 1994 August; 62(2): 269-72.
  http://www.ncbi.nlm.nih.gov:80/entrez/query.fcgi?cmd=Retrieve&db=PubMed&list_uids=8034071&dopt=Abstract

- **Prospective randomized study of human chorionic gonadotrophin priming before immature oocyte retrieval from unstimulated women with polycystic ovarian syndrome.**
  Author(s): Chian RC, Buckett WM, Tulandi T, Tan SL.
  Source: Human Reproduction (Oxford, England). 2000 January; 15(1): 165-70.
  http://www.ncbi.nlm.nih.gov:80/entrez/query.fcgi?cmd=Retrieve&db=PubMed&list_uids=10611207&dopt=Abstract

- **Puberty and polycystic ovarian syndrome: the insulin/insulin-like growth factor I hypothesis.**
  Author(s): Nobels F, Dewailly D.
  Source: Fertility and Sterility. 1992 October; 58(4): 655-66. Review.
  http://www.ncbi.nlm.nih.gov:80/entrez/query.fcgi?cmd=Retrieve&db=PubMed&list_uids=1426306&dopt=Abstract

- **Pulsatile luteinizing hormone-releasing hormone therapy in women with polycystic ovarian syndrome.**
  Author(s): Ory SJ.
  Source: Fertility and Sterility. 1988 June; 49(6): 941-3. Review.
  http://www.ncbi.nlm.nih.gov:80/entrez/query.fcgi?cmd=Retrieve&db=PubMed&list_uids=3131159&dopt=Abstract

- **Pulsatile secretion of serum gonadotropins in hirsute women with and without polycystic ovarian syndrome.**
  Author(s): Minanni SL, Wajchenberg BL, Marcondes JA, Cavaleiro-Luna AM, Fortes MA, Rego MA, Mendonca BB, Vezozzo DP, Rodbard D, Giannella-Neto D.
  Source: Annals of the New York Academy of Sciences. 1993 May 28; 687: 136-49.
  http://www.ncbi.nlm.nih.gov:80/entrez/query.fcgi?cmd=Retrieve&db=PubMed&list_uids=8323169&dopt=Abstract

- **Quantification of Doppler signal in polycystic ovarian syndrome using 3D power Doppler ultrasonography.**
  Author(s): Pan HA, Wu MH, Cheng YC, Li CH, Chang FM.
  Source: Human Reproduction (Oxford, England). 2002 September; 17(9): 2484.
  http://www.ncbi.nlm.nih.gov:80/entrez/query.fcgi?cmd=Retrieve&db=PubMed&list_uids=12202449&dopt=Abstract

- **Recurrent maternal virilization during pregnancy associated with polycystic ovarian syndrome: a case report and review of the literature.**
  Author(s): Ben-Chetrit A, Greenblatt EM.
  Source: Human Reproduction (Oxford, England). 1995 November; 10(11): 3057-60. Review.
  http://www.ncbi.nlm.nih.gov:80/entrez/query.fcgi?cmd=Retrieve&db=PubMed&list_uids=8747073&dopt=Abstract

- **Relationship between ultrasonography and histopathological changes in polycystic ovarian syndrome.**
  Author(s): Abdel Gadir A.
  Source: Human Reproduction (Oxford, England). 1995 July; 10(7): 1879.
  http://www.ncbi.nlm.nih.gov:80/entrez/query.fcgi?cmd=Retrieve&db=PubMed&list_uids=8583004&dopt=Abstract

- **Relationship between ultrasonography and histopathological changes in polycystic ovarian syndrome.**
  Author(s): Takahashi K, Ozaki T, Okada M, Uchida A, Kitao M.
  Source: Human Reproduction (Oxford, England). 1994 December; 9(12): 2255-8.
  http://www.ncbi.nlm.nih.gov:80/entrez/query.fcgi?cmd=Retrieve&db=PubMed&list_uids=7714140&dopt=Abstract

- **Relative risk of conversion from normoglycaemia to impaired glucose tolerance or non-insulin dependent diabetes mellitus in polycystic ovarian syndrome.**
  Author(s): Norman RJ, Masters L, Milner CR, Wang JX, Davies MJ.
  Source: Human Reproduction (Oxford, England). 2001 September; 16(9): 1995-8.
  http://www.ncbi.nlm.nih.gov:80/entrez/query.fcgi?cmd=Retrieve&db=PubMed&list_uids=11527911&dopt=Abstract

- **Relatively low levels of dimeric inhibin circulate in men and women with polycystic ovarian syndrome using a specific two-site enzyme-linked immunosorbent assay.**
  Author(s): Lambert-Messerlian GM, Hall JE, Sluss PM, Taylor AE, Martin KA, Groome NP, Crowley WF Jr, Schneyer AL.
  Source: The Journal of Clinical Endocrinology and Metabolism. 1994 July; 79(1): 45-50.
  http://www.ncbi.nlm.nih.gov:80/entrez/query.fcgi?cmd=Retrieve&db=PubMed&list_uids=8027251&dopt=Abstract

- **Response to clomiphene citrate in the polycystic ovarian syndrome according to different LH/FSH ratios.**
  Author(s): Lopez-Lopez E, Noguera MC, Fuente T, Parrilla JJ, Abad L.
  Source: Human Reproduction (Oxford, England). 1987 November; 2(8): 635-8.
  http://www.ncbi.nlm.nih.gov:80/entrez/query.fcgi?cmd=Retrieve&db=PubMed&list_uids=3125210&dopt=Abstract

- **Responses of polycystic ovarian syndrome and related variants to low-dose follicle stimulating hormone.**
    Author(s): Yong EL, Ng SC, Chan C, Kumar J, Teo LS, Ratnam S.
    Source: International Journal of Gynaecology and Obstetrics: the Official Organ of the International Federation of Gynaecology and Obstetrics. 1997 June; 57(3): 305-11.
    http://www.ncbi.nlm.nih.gov:80/entrez/query.fcgi?cmd=Retrieve&db=PubMed&list_uids=9215494&dopt=Abstract

- **Responses of somatostatin, beta-endorphin and dynorphin A to a glucose load in two groups of women with polycystic ovarian syndrome.**
    Author(s): Wu XK, Wang CH, Su YH.
    Source: Hormone Research. 1996; 46(2): 59-63.
    http://www.ncbi.nlm.nih.gov:80/entrez/query.fcgi?cmd=Retrieve&db=PubMed&list_uids=8871183&dopt=Abstract

- **Resting metabolic rate and postprandial thermogenesis in polycystic ovarian syndrome.**
    Author(s): Segal KR, Dunaif A.
    Source: Int J Obes. 1990 July; 14(7): 559-67.
    http://www.ncbi.nlm.nih.gov:80/entrez/query.fcgi?cmd=Retrieve&db=PubMed&list_uids=2228390&dopt=Abstract

- **Results of an open one-year study with Diane-35 in women with polycystic ovarian syndrome.**
    Author(s): Golland IM, Elstein ME.
    Source: Annals of the New York Academy of Sciences. 1993 May 28; 687: 263-71.
    http://www.ncbi.nlm.nih.gov:80/entrez/query.fcgi?cmd=Retrieve&db=PubMed&list_uids=8323182&dopt=Abstract

- **Resumption of ovarian function during lactational amenorrhoea in breastfeeding women with polycystic ovarian syndrome: endocrine aspects.**
    Author(s): Sir-Petermann T, Devoto L, Maliqueo M, Peirano P, Recabarren SE, Wildt L.
    Source: Human Reproduction (Oxford, England). 2001 August; 16(8): 1603-10.
    http://www.ncbi.nlm.nih.gov:80/entrez/query.fcgi?cmd=Retrieve&db=PubMed&list_uids=11473950&dopt=Abstract

- **Resumption of ovarian function during lactational amenorrhoea in breastfeeding women with polycystic ovarian syndrome: metabolic aspects.**
    Author(s): Maliqueo M, Sir-Petermann T, Salazar G, Perez-Bravo F, Recabarren SE, Wildt L.
    Source: Human Reproduction (Oxford, England). 2001 August; 16(8): 1598-602.
    http://www.ncbi.nlm.nih.gov:80/entrez/query.fcgi?cmd=Retrieve&db=PubMed&list_uids=11473949&dopt=Abstract

- **Role of growth hormone in polycystic ovarian syndrome.**
    Author(s): Morales AJ.
    Source: Semin Reprod Endocrinol. 1997 May; 15(2): 177-82. Review.
    http://www.ncbi.nlm.nih.gov:80/entrez/query.fcgi?cmd=Retrieve&db=PubMed&list_uids=9165661&dopt=Abstract

- **Secretory pattern of leptin and LH during lactational amenorrhoea in breastfeeding normal and polycystic ovarian syndrome women.**
  Author(s): Sir-Petermann T, Recabarren SE, Lobos A, Maliqueo M, Wildt L.
  Source: Human Reproduction (Oxford, England). 2001 February; 16(2): 244-9.
  http://www.ncbi.nlm.nih.gov:80/entrez/query.fcgi?cmd=Retrieve&db=PubMed&list_uids=11157814&dopt=Abstract

- **Sequential step-up and step-down dose regimen: an alternative method for ovulation induction with follicle-stimulating hormone in polycystic ovarian syndrome.**
  Author(s): Hugues JN, Cedrin-Durnerin I, Avril C, Bulwa S, Herve F, Uzan M.
  Source: Human Reproduction (Oxford, England). 1996 December; 11(12): 2581-4.
  http://www.ncbi.nlm.nih.gov:80/entrez/query.fcgi?cmd=Retrieve&db=PubMed&list_uids=9021354&dopt=Abstract

- **Serum luteinizing hormone profile during the menstrual cycle in polycystic ovarian syndrome.**
  Author(s): Minakami H, Abe N, Izumi A, Tamada T.
  Source: Fertility and Sterility. 1988 December; 50(6): 990-2.
  http://www.ncbi.nlm.nih.gov:80/entrez/query.fcgi?cmd=Retrieve&db=PubMed&list_uids=3060382&dopt=Abstract

- **Serum total renin is elevated in women with polycystic ovarian syndrome.**
  Author(s): Jaatinen TA, Matinlauri I, Anttila L, Koskinen P, Erkkola R, Irjala K.
  Source: Fertility and Sterility. 1995 May; 63(5): 1000-4.
  http://www.ncbi.nlm.nih.gov:80/entrez/query.fcgi?cmd=Retrieve&db=PubMed&list_uids=7720907&dopt=Abstract

- **Should patients with polycystic ovarian syndrome be treated with metformin?**
  Author(s): Seli E, Duleba AJ.
  Source: Human Reproduction (Oxford, England). 2002 September; 17(9): 2230-6. Review.
  http://www.ncbi.nlm.nih.gov:80/entrez/query.fcgi?cmd=Retrieve&db=PubMed&list_uids=12202407&dopt=Abstract

- **Should patients with polycystic ovarian syndrome be treated with metformin? A note of cautious optimism.**
  Author(s): Homburg R.
  Source: Human Reproduction (Oxford, England). 2002 April; 17(4): 853-6. Review.
  http://www.ncbi.nlm.nih.gov:80/entrez/query.fcgi?cmd=Retrieve&db=PubMed&list_uids=11925372&dopt=Abstract

- **Should patients with polycystic ovarian syndrome be treated with metformin?: an enthusiastic endorsement.**
  Author(s): Nestler JE.
  Source: Human Reproduction (Oxford, England). 2002 August; 17(8): 1950-3. Review.
  http://www.ncbi.nlm.nih.gov:80/entrez/query.fcgi?cmd=Retrieve&db=PubMed&list_uids=12151419&dopt=Abstract

- **Sonographic monitoring of ovarian volume during LHRH analogue therapy in women with polycystic ovarian syndrome.**
  Author(s): Jaffe R, Abramowicz J, Eckstein N, Vagman I, Fejgin M, Ayalon D.
  Source: Journal of Ultrasound in Medicine : Official Journal of the American Institute of Ultrasound in Medicine. 1988 April; 7(4): 203-6.
  http://www.ncbi.nlm.nih.gov:80/entrez/query.fcgi?cmd=Retrieve&db=PubMed&list_uids=2966864&dopt=Abstract

- **Specific factors predict the response to pulsatile gonadotropin-releasing hormone therapy in polycystic ovarian syndrome.**
  Author(s): Gill S, Taylor AE, Martin KA, Welt CK, Adams JM, Hall JE.
  Source: The Journal of Clinical Endocrinology and Metabolism. 2001 June; 86(6): 2428-36.
  http://www.ncbi.nlm.nih.gov:80/entrez/query.fcgi?cmd=Retrieve&db=PubMed&list_uids=11397835&dopt=Abstract

- **Stimulation with human menopausal gonadotropin versus follicle-stimulating hormone after pituitary suppression in polycystic ovarian syndrome.**
  Author(s): Tanbo T, Dale PO, Kjekshus E, Haug E, Abyholm T.
  Source: Fertility and Sterility. 1990 May; 53(5): 798-803.
  http://www.ncbi.nlm.nih.gov:80/entrez/query.fcgi?cmd=Retrieve&db=PubMed&list_uids=2110071&dopt=Abstract

- **Successful delivery following cryopreservation of zygotes produced by in vitro matured oocytes retrieved from a woman with polycystic ovarian syndrome-like disease: a case report.**
  Author(s): Kyono K, Fukunaga N, Haigo K, Chiba S, Ohira C, Nakajo Y, Araki Y.
  Source: Journal of Assisted Reproduction and Genetics. 2002 August; 19(8): 390-3.
  http://www.ncbi.nlm.nih.gov:80/entrez/query.fcgi?cmd=Retrieve&db=PubMed&list_uids=12182446&dopt=Abstract

- **Suppression of serum prolactin levels after an oral glucose tolerance test in patients with polycystic ovarian syndrome.**
  Author(s): Rousso D, Skiadopoulos S, Rousso I, Kalahanis J, Petropoulos P, Mavromatidis G, Panidis D.
  Source: Gynecologic and Obstetric Investigation. 1997; 44(2): 120-3.
  http://www.ncbi.nlm.nih.gov:80/entrez/query.fcgi?cmd=Retrieve&db=PubMed&list_uids=9286726&dopt=Abstract

- **Surgical management of polycystic ovarian syndrome.**
  Author(s): Tulandi T, al Took S.
  Source: Baillieres Clin Obstet Gynaecol. 1998 December; 12(4): 541-53. Review.
  http://www.ncbi.nlm.nih.gov:80/entrez/query.fcgi?cmd=Retrieve&db=PubMed&list_uids=10627766&dopt=Abstract

- **Tamoxifen: an alternative approach in clomiphene resistant polycystic ovarian syndrome patients.**
  Author(s): Gulekli B, Ozaksit G, Turhan NO, Senoz S, Oral H, Gokmen O.
  Source: J Pak Med Assoc. 1993 May; 43(5): 89-90.
  http://www.ncbi.nlm.nih.gov:80/entrez/query.fcgi?cmd=Retrieve&db=PubMed&list_uids=8264082&dopt=Abstract

- **Temporal lobe epilepsy: an extrahypothalamic pathogenesis for polycystic ovarian syndrome?**
  Author(s): Herzog AG, Seibel MM, Schomer D, Vaitukaitis J, Geschwind N.
  Source: Neurology. 1984 October; 34(10): 1389-93.
  http://www.ncbi.nlm.nih.gov:80/entrez/query.fcgi?cmd=Retrieve&db=PubMed&list_uids=6541317&dopt=Abstract

- **The acute effects of a dopamine antagonist (domperidone) on luteinising hormone, follicle stimulating hormone, prolactin and thyrotrophin secretion in polycystic ovarian syndrome: differential effect of ovulation.**
  Author(s): Murdoch AP, Dunlop W, Kendall-Taylor P, Watson MJ.
  Source: Clinical Endocrinology. 1984 December; 21(6): 611-9.
  http://www.ncbi.nlm.nih.gov:80/entrez/query.fcgi?cmd=Retrieve&db=PubMed&list_uids=6439439&dopt=Abstract

- **The behavior of follicle cysts formed after long-acting gonadotropin-releasing hormone analog administration in patients with polycystic ovarian syndrome.**
  Author(s): Ellenbogen A, Abu-Asbah I, Libal Y, Jaschevatzky O, Anderman S, Ballas S.
  Source: Gynecological Endocrinology : the Official Journal of the International Society of Gynecological Endocrinology. 1997 April; 11(2): 101-4.
  http://www.ncbi.nlm.nih.gov:80/entrez/query.fcgi?cmd=Retrieve&db=PubMed&list_uids=9174850&dopt=Abstract

- **The biological variation of insulin resistance in polycystic ovarian syndrome.**
  Author(s): Jayagopal V, Kilpatrick ES, Holding S, Jennings PE, Atkin SL.
  Source: The Journal of Clinical Endocrinology and Metabolism. 2002 April; 87(4): 1560-2.
  http://www.ncbi.nlm.nih.gov:80/entrez/query.fcgi?cmd=Retrieve&db=PubMed&list_uids=11932282&dopt=Abstract

- **The biological variation of testosterone and sex hormone-binding globulin (SHBG) in polycystic ovarian syndrome: implications for SHBG as a surrogate marker of insulin resistance.**
  Author(s): Jayagopal V, Kilpatrick ES, Jennings PE, Hepburn DA, Atkin SL.
  Source: The Journal of Clinical Endocrinology and Metabolism. 2003 April; 88(4): 1528-33.
  http://www.ncbi.nlm.nih.gov:80/entrez/query.fcgi?cmd=Retrieve&db=PubMed&list_uids=12679434&dopt=Abstract

- **The chromosomal normality of unfertilized oocytes from patients with polycystic ovarian syndrome.**
  Author(s): Sengoku K, Tamate K, Takuma N, Yoshida T, Goishi K, Ishikawa M.
  Source: Human Reproduction (Oxford, England). 1997 March; 12(3): 474-7.
  http://www.ncbi.nlm.nih.gov:80/entrez/query.fcgi?cmd=Retrieve&db=PubMed&list_uids=9130743&dopt=Abstract

- **The course and outcome of pregnancy after ovarian electrocautery in women with polycystic ovarian syndrome: the influence of body-weight.**
  Author(s): Gjonnaess H.
  Source: British Journal of Obstetrics and Gynaecology. 1989 June; 96(6): 714-9.
  http://www.ncbi.nlm.nih.gov:80/entrez/query.fcgi?cmd=Retrieve&db=PubMed&list_uids=2803993&dopt=Abstract

- **The effect of gonadotropin-releasing hormone agonist on the ovarian response and in vitro fertilization results in polycystic ovarian syndrome: a prospective study.**
  Author(s): Dor J, Shulman A, Pariente C, Levran D, Bider D, Menashe Y, Mashiach S.
  Source: Fertility and Sterility. 1992 February; 57(2): 366-71.
  http://www.ncbi.nlm.nih.gov:80/entrez/query.fcgi?cmd=Retrieve&db=PubMed&list_uids=1531200&dopt=Abstract

- **The effect of metoclopramide on ovarian responsiveness to gonadotropin administration in patients with severe polycystic ovarian syndrome.**
  Author(s): Lissak A, Dirnfeld M, Sorokin Y, Kahana L, Abramovici H, Koch Y.
  Source: Fertility and Sterility. 1990 October; 54(4): 585-9.
  http://www.ncbi.nlm.nih.gov:80/entrez/query.fcgi?cmd=Retrieve&db=PubMed&list_uids=2209878&dopt=Abstract

- **The entero-insular axis in polycystic ovarian syndrome.**
  Author(s): Gama R, Norris F, Wright J, Morgan L, Hampton S, Watkins S, Marks V.
  Source: Annals of Clinical Biochemistry. 1996 May; 33 (Pt 3): 190-5.
  http://www.ncbi.nlm.nih.gov:80/entrez/query.fcgi?cmd=Retrieve&db=PubMed&list_uids=8791980&dopt=Abstract

- **The impact of ethnicity on the presentation of polycystic ovarian syndrome.**
  Author(s): Williamson K, Gunn AJ, Johnson N, Milsom SR.
  Source: The Australian & New Zealand Journal of Obstetrics & Gynaecology. 2001 May; 41(2): 202-6.
  http://www.ncbi.nlm.nih.gov:80/entrez/query.fcgi?cmd=Retrieve&db=PubMed&list_uids=11453273&dopt=Abstract

- **The impact of obesity and insulin resistance on the outcome of IVF or ICSI in women with polycystic ovarian syndrome.**
  Author(s): Fedorcsak P, Dale PO, Storeng R, Tanbo T, Abyholm T.
  Source: Human Reproduction (Oxford, England). 2001 June; 16(6): 1086-91.
  http://www.ncbi.nlm.nih.gov:80/entrez/query.fcgi?cmd=Retrieve&db=PubMed&list_uids=11387273&dopt=Abstract

- **The influence of body mass index, basal FSH and age on the response to gonadotrophin stimulation in non-polycystic ovarian syndrome patients.**
  Author(s): Loh S, Wang JX, Matthews CD.
  Source: Human Reproduction (Oxford, England). 2002 May; 17(5): 1207-11.
  http://www.ncbi.nlm.nih.gov:80/entrez/query.fcgi?cmd=Retrieve&db=PubMed&list_uids=11980739&dopt=Abstract

- **The influence of luteinizing hormone and insulin on sex steroids and sex hormone-binding globulin in the polycystic ovarian syndrome.**
  Author(s): Buyalos RP, Geffner ME, Watanabe RM, Bergman RN, Gornbein JA, Judd HL.
  Source: Fertility and Sterility. 1993 October; 60(4): 626-33.
  http://www.ncbi.nlm.nih.gov:80/entrez/query.fcgi?cmd=Retrieve&db=PubMed&list_uids=8405515&dopt=Abstract

- **The number of follicles and ovarian volume in the assessment of response to clomiphene citrate treatment in polycystic ovarian syndrome.**
  Author(s): Ficicioglu C, Api M, Ozden S.
  Source: Acta Obstetricia Et Gynecologica Scandinavica. 1996 November; 75(10): 917-21.
  http://www.ncbi.nlm.nih.gov:80/entrez/query.fcgi?cmd=Retrieve&db=PubMed&list_uids=9003093&dopt=Abstract

- **The number of follicles and ovarian volume in the assessment of the response to clomiphene citrate in polycystic ovarian syndrome.**
  Author(s): Ficicioglu C, Api M, Ozden S.
  Source: Acta Eur Fertil. 1995 May-June; 26(3): 101-4.
  http://www.ncbi.nlm.nih.gov:80/entrez/query.fcgi?cmd=Retrieve&db=PubMed&list_uids=9098468&dopt=Abstract

- **The ovarian renin-angiotensin system in polycystic ovarian syndrome.**
  Author(s): Palumbo A, Carcangiu ML, Roa L, Pepperell J, Pourmotabbed G, Naftolin F.
  Source: Annals of the New York Academy of Sciences. 1993 May 28; 687: 39-45. Review.
  http://www.ncbi.nlm.nih.gov:80/entrez/query.fcgi?cmd=Retrieve&db=PubMed&list_uids=8323188&dopt=Abstract

- **The prognostic value of basal luteinizing hormone:follicle-stimulating hormone ratio in the treatment of patients with polycystic ovarian syndrome by assisted reproduction techniques.**
  Author(s): Tarlatzis BC, Grimbizis G, Pournaropoulos F, Bontis J, Lagos S, Spanos E, Mantalenakis S.
  Source: Human Reproduction (Oxford, England). 1995 October; 10(10): 2545-9.
  http://www.ncbi.nlm.nih.gov:80/entrez/query.fcgi?cmd=Retrieve&db=PubMed&list_uids=8567767&dopt=Abstract

- **The relation between obesity and testosterone-estradiol binding globulin levels in polycystic ovarian syndrome (PCO).**
  Author(s): Badawy SZ, Weigert JM, Marshall LD, Cuenca VG.
  Source: Diagn Gynecol Obstet. 1980 Spring; 2(1): 43-6.
  http://www.ncbi.nlm.nih.gov:80/entrez/query.fcgi?cmd=Retrieve&db=PubMed&list_uids=7193560&dopt=Abstract

- **The relation of the gonadotrophin response to chlormadinone according to body weight in patients with amenorrhea due to polycystic ovarian syndrome.**
  Author(s): Carranza-Lira S, Garcia-Hernandez E, Baiza MR, Moran C.
  Source: European Journal of Obstetrics, Gynecology, and Reproductive Biology. 1996 June; 66(2): 161-4.
  http://www.ncbi.nlm.nih.gov:80/entrez/query.fcgi?cmd=Retrieve&db=PubMed&list_uids=8735740&dopt=Abstract

- **The relationship between circulating androgens, obesity, and hyperinsulinemia on serum insulin-like growth factor binding protein-1 in the polycystic ovarian syndrome.**
  Author(s): Buyalos RP, Pekonen F, Halme JK, Judd HL, Rutanen EM.
  Source: American Journal of Obstetrics and Gynecology. 1995 March; 172(3): 932-9.
  http://www.ncbi.nlm.nih.gov:80/entrez/query.fcgi?cmd=Retrieve&db=PubMed&list_uids=7534449&dopt=Abstract

- **The response of the growth hormone and insulin-like growth factor I axis to medical castration in women with polycystic ovarian syndrome.**
  Author(s): Hatasaka HH, Kazer RR, Chatterton RT, Unterman TG, Glick RP.
  Source: Fertility and Sterility. 1994 August; 62(2): 273-8.
  http://www.ncbi.nlm.nih.gov:80/entrez/query.fcgi?cmd=Retrieve&db=PubMed&list_uids=8034072&dopt=Abstract

- **The role of adrenal hyperandrogenism, insulin resistance, and obesity in the pathogenesis of polycystic ovarian syndrome.**
  Author(s): Rittmaster RS, Deshwal N, Lehman L.
  Source: The Journal of Clinical Endocrinology and Metabolism. 1993 May; 76(5): 1295-300.
  http://www.ncbi.nlm.nih.gov:80/entrez/query.fcgi?cmd=Retrieve&db=PubMed&list_uids=8388405&dopt=Abstract

- **The role of computed tomography in the diagnosis of polycystic ovarian syndrome.**
  Author(s): Al Mahallawi MN, Al Ahwani S, Jeanmart E.
  Source: J Belge Radiol. 1984; 67(2): 81-5. No Abstract Available.
  http://www.ncbi.nlm.nih.gov:80/entrez/query.fcgi?cmd=Retrieve&db=PubMed&list_uids=6490591&dopt=Abstract

- **The role of neurotransmitters and opioids in polycystic ovarian syndrome.**
  Author(s): Lobo RA.
  Source: Endocrinology and Metabolism Clinics of North America. 1988 December; 17(4): 667-83. Review.
  http://www.ncbi.nlm.nih.gov:80/entrez/query.fcgi?cmd=Retrieve&db=PubMed&list_uids=2904366&dopt=Abstract

- **The significance of high follicular-phase luteinizing hormone levels in the treatment of women with polycystic ovarian syndrome by in vitro fertilization.**
  Author(s): Tarlatzis BC, Grimbizis G.
  Source: Journal of Assisted Reproduction and Genetics. 1997 January; 14(1): 1-4. Review.
  http://www.ncbi.nlm.nih.gov:80/entrez/query.fcgi?cmd=Retrieve&db=PubMed&list_uids=9013299&dopt=Abstract

- **'The thief of womanhood': women's experience of polycystic ovarian syndrome.**
  Author(s): Kitzinger C, Willmott J.
  Source: Social Science & Medicine (1982). 2002 February; 54(3): 349-61.
  http://www.ncbi.nlm.nih.gov:80/entrez/query.fcgi?cmd=Retrieve&db=PubMed&list_uids=11824912&dopt=Abstract

- **The treatment of patients with polycystic ovarian syndrome by in-vitro fertilization and embryo transfer: a comparison of results with those of patients with tubal infertility.**
  Author(s): Dor J, Shulman A, Levran D, Ben-Rafael Z, Rudak E, Mashiach S.
  Source: Human Reproduction (Oxford, England). 1990 October; 5(7): 816-8.
  http://www.ncbi.nlm.nih.gov:80/entrez/query.fcgi?cmd=Retrieve&db=PubMed&list_uids=2266154&dopt=Abstract

- **Therapeutic use of gonadotropin-releasing hormone agonists in polycystic ovarian syndrome.**
  Author(s): Markussis V, Goni MH, Tolis G.
  Source: Annals of the New York Academy of Sciences. 1993 May 28; 687: 242-9. Review.
  http://www.ncbi.nlm.nih.gov:80/entrez/query.fcgi?cmd=Retrieve&db=PubMed&list_uids=8323179&dopt=Abstract

- **Three types of polycystic ovarian syndrome in relation to androgenic function.**
  Author(s): Takai I, Taii S, Takakura K, Mori T.
  Source: Fertility and Sterility. 1991 November; 56(5): 856-62.
  http://www.ncbi.nlm.nih.gov:80/entrez/query.fcgi?cmd=Retrieve&db=PubMed&list_uids=1936318&dopt=Abstract

- **Three-dimensional assessment of ultrasound features in women with clomiphene citrate-resistant polycystic ovarian syndrome (PCOS): ovarian stromal volume does not correlate with biochemical indices.**
  Author(s): Nardo LG, Buckett WM, White D, Digesu AG, Franks S, Khullar V.
  Source: Human Reproduction (Oxford, England). 2002 April; 17(4): 1052-5.
  http://www.ncbi.nlm.nih.gov:80/entrez/query.fcgi?cmd=Retrieve&db=PubMed&list_uids=11925404&dopt=Abstract

- **Transitional cell carcinoma of the bladder in a young woman with the polycystic ovarian syndrome.**
  Author(s): Scott MJ, Parkhouse H, Hendry WF.
  Source: British Journal of Urology. 1993 February; 71(2): 235.
  http://www.ncbi.nlm.nih.gov:80/entrez/query.fcgi?cmd=Retrieve&db=PubMed&list_uids=8461963&dopt=Abstract

- **Transvaginal ultrasonic assessment of the response to clomiphene citrate in polycystic ovarian syndrome.**
  Author(s): Takahashi K, Uchida A, Yamasaki H, Ozaki T, Kitao M.
  Source: Fertility and Sterility. 1994 July; 62(1): 48-53.
  http://www.ncbi.nlm.nih.gov:80/entrez/query.fcgi?cmd=Retrieve&db=PubMed&list_uids=8005303&dopt=Abstract

- **Transvaginal ultrasonographic morphology in polycystic ovarian syndrome.**
  Author(s): Takahashi K, Okada M, Ozaki T, Uchida A, Yamasaki H, Kitao M.
  Source: Gynecologic and Obstetric Investigation. 1995; 39(3): 201-6.
  http://www.ncbi.nlm.nih.gov:80/entrez/query.fcgi?cmd=Retrieve&db=PubMed&list_uids=7789918&dopt=Abstract

- **Transvaginal ultrasound imaging, histopathology and endocrinopathy in patients with polycystic ovarian syndrome.**
  Author(s): Takahashi K, Eda Y, Abu-Musa A, Okada S, Yoshino K, Kitao M.
  Source: Human Reproduction (Oxford, England). 1994 July; 9(7): 1231-6.
  http://www.ncbi.nlm.nih.gov:80/entrez/query.fcgi?cmd=Retrieve&db=PubMed&list_uids=7962423&dopt=Abstract

- **Treatment in polycystic ovarian syndrome (PCOS) with emphasis on ovarian electrocautery.**
  Author(s): Gjonnaess H.
  Source: Ginekol Pol. 1998 December; 69(12): 855-8. Review.
  http://www.ncbi.nlm.nih.gov:80/entrez/query.fcgi?cmd=Retrieve&db=PubMed&list_uids=10224741&dopt=Abstract

- **Treatment of anovulation due to polycystic ovarian syndrome by laparoscopic ovarian electrocautery.**
  Author(s): Kovacs G, Buckler H, Bangah M, Outch K, Burger H, Healy D, Baker G, Phillips S.
  Source: British Journal of Obstetrics and Gynaecology. 1991 January; 98(1): 30-5.
  http://www.ncbi.nlm.nih.gov:80/entrez/query.fcgi?cmd=Retrieve&db=PubMed&list_uids=1825605&dopt=Abstract

- **Treatment of clomiphene citrate-resistant polycystic ovarian syndrome with pure follicle-stimulating hormone or human menopausal gonadotropin.**
  Author(s): McFaul PB, Traub AI, Thompson W.
  Source: Fertility and Sterility. 1990 May; 53(5): 792-7.
  http://www.ncbi.nlm.nih.gov:80/entrez/query.fcgi?cmd=Retrieve&db=PubMed&list_uids=2110070&dopt=Abstract

- **Treatment of the infertile patient with polycystic ovarian syndrome.**
  Author(s): Pritts EA.
  Source: Obstetrical & Gynecological Survey. 2002 September; 57(9): 587-97. Review.
  http://www.ncbi.nlm.nih.gov:80/entrez/query.fcgi?cmd=Retrieve&db=PubMed&list_uids=12218667&dopt=Abstract

- **Ultrasound-detected polycystic ovarian syndrome associated with depleted basal level but enhanced response of gonadotropin.**
  Author(s): Imai A, Furui T, Tamaya T.
  Source: J Med. 1995; 26(5-6): 337-42.
  http://www.ncbi.nlm.nih.gov:80/entrez/query.fcgi?cmd=Retrieve&db=PubMed&list_uids=8721909&dopt=Abstract

- **Vaginal progesterone administration before ovulation induction with exogenous gonadotropins in polycystic ovarian syndrome.**
  Author(s): Buckler HM, Phillips SE, Cameron IT, Healy DL, Burger HG.
  Source: The Journal of Clinical Endocrinology and Metabolism. 1988 August; 67(2): 300-6.
  http://www.ncbi.nlm.nih.gov:80/entrez/query.fcgi?cmd=Retrieve&db=PubMed&list_uids=3134388&dopt=Abstract

- **Vaginal progesterone administration in physiological doses normalizes raised luteinizing hormone levels in patients with polycystic ovarian syndrome.**
  Author(s): Buckler HM, Bangah M, Healy DL, Burger HG.
  Source: Gynecological Endocrinology : the Official Journal of the International Society of Gynecological Endocrinology. 1992 December; 6(4): 275-82.
  http://www.ncbi.nlm.nih.gov:80/entrez/query.fcgi?cmd=Retrieve&db=PubMed&list_uids=1492584&dopt=Abstract

- **Valproate and the polycystic ovarian syndrome: final thoughts.**
  Author(s): Herzog AG, Schachter SC.
  Source: Epilepsia. 2001 March; 42(3): 311-5.
  http://www.ncbi.nlm.nih.gov:80/entrez/query.fcgi?cmd=Retrieve&db=PubMed&list_uids=11442145&dopt=Abstract

- **Valproate, bipolar disorder and polycystic ovarian syndrome.**
  Author(s): McIntyre RS, Mancini DA, McCann S, Srinivasan J, Kennedy SH.
  Source: Bipolar Disorders. 2003 February; 5(1): 28-35.
  http://www.ncbi.nlm.nih.gov:80/entrez/query.fcgi?cmd=Retrieve&db=PubMed&list_uids=12656935&dopt=Abstract

- **Vitamin D and calcium dysregulation in the polycystic ovarian syndrome.**
  Author(s): Thys-Jacobs S, Donovan D, Papadopoulos A, Sarrel P, Bilezikian JP.
  Source: Steroids. 1999 June; 64(6): 430-5.
  http://www.ncbi.nlm.nih.gov:80/entrez/query.fcgi?cmd=Retrieve&db=PubMed&list_uids=10433180&dopt=Abstract

- **What is polycystic ovarian syndrome? A proposal for a consensus on the definition and diagnosis of polycystic ovarian syndrome.**
  Author(s): Homburg R.
  Source: Human Reproduction (Oxford, England). 2002 October; 17(10): 2495-9. Review.
  http://www.ncbi.nlm.nih.gov:80/entrez/query.fcgi?cmd=Retrieve&db=PubMed&list_uids=12351518&dopt=Abstract

CHAPTER 2. NUTRITION AND POLYCYSTIC OVARIAN SYNDROME

Overview

In this chapter, we will show you how to find studies dedicated specifically to nutrition and polycystic ovarian syndrome.

Finding Nutrition Studies on Polycystic Ovarian Syndrome

The National Institutes of Health's Office of Dietary Supplements (ODS) offers a searchable bibliographic database called the IBIDS (International Bibliographic Information on Dietary Supplements; National Institutes of Health, Building 31, Room 1B29, 31 Center Drive, MSC 2086, Bethesda, Maryland 20892-2086, Tel: 301-435-2920, Fax: 301-480-1845, E-mail: ods@nih.gov). The IBIDS contains over 460,000 scientific citations and summaries about dietary supplements and nutrition as well as references to published international, scientific literature on dietary supplements such as vitamins, minerals, and botanicals.[7] The IBIDS includes references and citations to both human and animal research studies.

As a service of the ODS, access to the IBIDS database is available free of charge at the following Web address: **http://ods.od.nih.gov/databases/ibids.html**. After entering the search area, you have three choices: (1) IBIDS Consumer Database, (2) Full IBIDS Database, or (3) Peer Reviewed Citations Only.

Now that you have selected a database, click on the "Advanced" tab. An advanced search allows you to retrieve up to 100 fully explained references in a comprehensive format. Type "polycystic ovarian syndrome" (or synonyms) into the search box, and click "Go." To narrow the search, you can also select the "Title" field.

---

[7] Adapted from **http://ods.od.nih.gov**. IBIDS is produced by the Office of Dietary Supplements (ODS) at the National Institutes of Health to assist the public, healthcare providers, educators, and researchers in locating credible, scientific information on dietary supplements. IBIDS was developed and will be maintained through an interagency partnership with the Food and Nutrition Information Center of the National Agricultural Library, U.S. Department of Agriculture.

The following information is typical of that found when using the "Full IBIDS Database" to search for "polycystic ovarian syndrome" (or a synonym):

- **A comparative study of fixed-dose, step-down, and low-dose step-up regimens of human menopausal gonadotropin for patients with polycystic ovary syndrome.**
  Author(s): Department of Obstetrics and Gynecology, Gunma University School of Medicine, Maebashi, Japan.
  Source: Andoh, K Mizunuma, H Liu, X Kamijo, T Yamada, K Ibuki, Y Fertil-Steril. 1998 November; 70(5): 840-6 0015-0282

- **A randomized controlled study comparing the endocrine effects of pulsatile intravenous gonadotropin-releasing hormone after gonadotropin-releasing hormone agonist pretreatment versus clomiphene citrate in patients with polycystic ovary syndrome.**
  Author(s): Catharina Hospital, Eindhoven, The Netherlands.
  Source: Timmerman van Kessel, E C Cikot, R J Dargel Donkers, E J Zwertbroek, W van Dop, P A Schoot, D C Fertil-Steril. 2000 June; 73(6): 1145-8 0015-0282

- **Adrenal dynamic responses to physiologic and pharmacologic adrenocorticotropic hormone stimulation before and after ovarian steroid modulation in women with polycystic ovary syndrome.**
  Author(s): Department of Gynecology and Obstetrics, School of Medicine and Biomedical Sciences, State University of New York at Buffalo, USA.
  Source: Gonzalez, F Chang, L Horab, T Stanczyk, F Z Crickard, K Lobo, R A Fertil-Steril. 1999 March; 71(3): 439-44 0015-0282

- **Attenuation of ovarian response by low-dose ketoconazole during superovulation in patients with polycystic ovary syndrome.**
  Author(s): Shaare Zedek Medical Center, The Alexander Silberman Institute of Life Sciences, The Hebrew University of Jerusalem, Israel. gal_m@netvision.net.il
  Source: Gal, M Eldar Geva, T Margalioth, E J Barr, I Orly, J Diamant, Y Z Fertil-Steril. 1999 July; 72(1): 26-31 0015-0282

- **Cabergoline influences ovarian stimulation in hyperprolactinaemic patients with polycystic ovary syndrome.**
  Author(s): Department of Obstetrics and Gynecology, San Raffaele Scientific Institute, University of Milan, Italy. enrypap@hotmail.com
  Source: Papaleo, E Doldi, N De Santis, L Marelli, G Marsiglio, E Rofena, S Ferrari, A Hum-Reprod. 2001 November; 16(11): 2263-6 0268-1161

- **Clomiphene citrate-resistant polycystic ovary syndrome. Preventing multifollicular development.**
  Author(s): Department of Obstetrics and Gynecology, Gulhane Military Medical Academy, Istanbul, Turkey.
  Source: Ergur, A R Yergok, Y Z Ertekin, A Kucuk, T Mungen, E Tutuncu, L J-Reprod-Med. 1998 March; 43(3): 185-90 0024-7758

- **Co-administration of metformin during rFSH treatment in patients with clomiphene citrate-resistant polycystic ovarian syndrome: a prospective randomized trial.**
  Author(s): Department of Obstetrics and Gynecology, Division of Reproductive Endocrinology and Infertility, Hacettepe University, Ankara, Turkey. yarali@ada.net.tr
  Source: Yarali, Hakan Yildiz, Bulent O Demirol, Aygul Zeyneloglu, Hulusi B Yigit, Nuray Bukulmez, Orhan Koray, Zehra Hum-Reprod. 2002 February; 17(2): 289-94 0268-1161

- **Cohort size rather than follicle-stimulating hormone threshold level determines ovarian sensitivity in polycystic ovary syndrome.**
  Author(s): Department of Obstetrics and Gynaecology, University Hospital Vrije Universiteit, Amsterdam, The Netherlands.
  Source: Van Der Meer, M Hompes, P G De Boer, J A Schats, R Schoemaker, J J-Clin-Endocrinol-Metab. 1998 February; 83(2): 423-6 0021-972X

- **Combined somatostatin analog and follicle-stimulating hormone for women with polycystic ovary syndrome resistant to conventional treatment.**
  Author(s): Department of Obstetrics and Gynecology, Chaim Sheba Medical Center, Tel Hashomer, Israel.
  Source: Lidor, A Soriano, D Seidman, D S Dor, J Mashiach, S Rabinovici, J Gynecol-Endocrinol. 1998 April; 12(2): 97-101 0951-3590

- **Dexamethasone supplementation to gonadotropin stimulation for in vitro fertilization in polycystic ovarian disease.**
  Author(s): Department of Obstetrics and Gynecology, Chaim Sheba Medical Center, Tel Hashomer, Israel.
  Source: Bider, D Hourvitz, A Tur Kaspa, I Dirnfeld, M Dor, J J-Assist-Reprod-Genet. 1999 May; 16(5): 233-5 1058-0468

- **'Early coasting' in patients with polycystic ovarian syndrome is consistent with good clinical outcome.**
  Author(s): IVF Centre, Maternity Hospital, Kuwait.
  Source: Egbase, P E Al Sharhan, M Grudzinskas, J G Hum-Reprod. 2002 May; 17(5): 1212-6 0268-1161

- **Effect of gonadotrophin-releasing hormone agonist treatment on growth hormone secretion in women with polycystic ovarian syndrome.**
  Author(s): Endocrine Clinic, PANAGIA Hospital, Thessaloniki, Greece.
  Source: Kaltsas, T Pontikides, N Krassas, G E Seferiadis, K Lolis, D Messinis, I E Hum-Reprod. 1998 January; 13(1): 22-6 0268-1161

- **Evaluation and therapy of polycystic ovarian syndrome.**
  Author(s): Department of Obstetrics and Gynecology, Harvard Medical School, Beth Israel Hospital, Boston, Massachusetts.
  Source: Loy, R Seibel, M M Endocrinol-Metab-Clin-North-Am. 1988 December; 17(4): 785-813 0889-8529

- **Evaluation of ovarian cysts following GnRH-a treatment in patients with polycystic ovarian syndrome.**
  Author(s): Second Department of Obstetrics and Gynecology, University of Athens, Areteion Hospital, Athens, Greece.
  Source: Gregoriou, O Vitoratos, N Konidaris, S Papadias, C Chryssikopoulos, A Gynecol-Obstet-Invest. 1998; 46(4): 252-5 0378-7346

- **Follistatin and activin A serum concentrations in obese and non-obese patients with polycystic ovary syndrome.**
  Author(s): IVF Unit and Institute for Hormone Research, Shaare-Zedek Medical Center, Ben-Gurion University, P.O. Box 3235, Jerusalem, Israel. gevat@szmc.org.il
  Source: Eldar Geva, T Spitz, I M Groome, N P Margalioth, E J Homburg, R Hum-Reprod. 2001 December; 16(12): 2552-6 0268-1161

- **Gonadotrophin therapy for ovulation induction in subfertility associated with polycystic ovary syndrome.**
  Author(s): Assisted Conception Unit, Clarendon Wing, Leeds General Infirmary, Clarendon Road, Leeds, UK, LS1 3EX. d.nugent@leeds.ac.uk
  Source: Nugent, D Vandekerckhove, P Hughes, E Arnot, M Lilford, R Cochrane-Database-Syst-Revolume 2000; (4): CD000410 1469-493X

- **Gonadotrophin-releasing hormone analogue as an adjunct to gonadotropin therapy for clomiphene-resistant polycystic ovarian syndrome.**
  Author(s): Rm HSC-4F7, Department of Obstetrics and Gynaecology, McMaster University, 1200 Main St West, Hamilton, Ontario, Canada, L8N 3Z5. hughese@fhs.csu.mcmaster.ca
  Source: Hughes, E Collins, J Vandekerckhove, P Cochrane-Database-Syst-Revolume 2000; (2): CD000097 1469-493X

- **Growth hormone response to thyrotrophin releasing hormone in women with polycystic ovarian syndrome.**
  Author(s): Department of Endocrinology, PANAGIA Hospital, Thessaloniki, Greece.
  Source: Kaltsas, T Pontikides, N Krassas, G E Seferiadis, K Lolis, D Messinis, I E Hum-Reprod. 1999 November; 14(11): 2704-8 0268-1161

- **Increased 5alpha-reductase and normal 11beta-hydroxysteroid dehydrogenase metabolism of C19 and C21 steroids in a young population with polycystic ovarian syndrome.**
  Author(s): Department of Pediatrics, New York University Medical Center, New York, USA.
  Source: Chin, D Shackleton, C Prasad, V K Kohn, B David, R Imperato McGinley, J Cohen, H McMahon, D J Oberfield, S E J-Pediatr-Endocrinol-Metab. 2000 March; 13(3): 253-9

- **Induction of ovulation by pulsatile LH-RH administration in polycystic ovarian syndrome.**
  Source: Bolanowski, M Grabinski, M Milewicz, A Zalewski, J Endokrynol-Pol. 1989; 40(6): 281-4 0423-104X

- **Inhibin A and inhibin B in women with polycystic ovarian syndrome during treatment with FSH to induce mono-ovulation.**
  Author(s): Department of Obstetrics and Gynaecology, University of Edinburgh, UK.
  Source: Anderson, R A Groome, N P Baird, D T Clin-Endocrinol-(Oxf). 1998 May; 48(5): 577-84 0300-0664

- **Insulin and C-peptide secretion in non-obese patients with polycystic ovarian disease.**
  Author(s): Department of Chemical Pathology, University of Natal Medical School, Durban, Republic of South Africa.
  Source: Mahabeer, S Jialal, I Norman, R J Naidoo, C Reddi, K Joubert, S M Horm-Metab-Res. 1989 September; 21(9): 502-6 0018-5043

- **Insulin stimulates testosterone biosynthesis by human thecal cells from women with polycystic ovary syndrome by activating its own receptor and using inositolglycan mediators as the signal transduction system.**
  Author(s): Department of Internal Medicine, Medical College of Virginia/Virginia Commonwealth University, Richmond 23298, USA. nestler@hsc.vcu.edu
  Source: Nestler, J E Jakubowicz, D J de Vargas, A F Brik, C Quintero, N Medina, F J-Clin-Endocrinol-Metab. 1998 June; 83(6): 2001-5 0021-972X

- **Lack of insulin-like growth factor binding protein-3 variation after follicle-stimulating hormone stimulation in women with polycystic ovary syndrome undergoing in vitro fertilization.**
  Author(s): Department of Endocrinology, Second University of Naples, Italy.
  Source: Amato, G Izzo, A Tucker, A T Bellastella, A Fertil-Steril. 1999 September; 72(3): 454-7 0015-0282

- **Limited ovarian stimulation results in the recovery of mature oocytes in polycystic ovarian disease patients: a preliminary report.**
  Author(s): Al Salama Hospital IVF Unit, Jeddah, Saudi Arabia.
  Source: El Sheikh, M M Hussein, M Sheikh, A A Fouad, S El Sheikh, R Al Hasani, S Eur-J-Obstet-Gynecol-Reprod-Biol. 1999 March; 83(1): 81-3 0301-2115

- **Low-dose FSH stimulation in polycystic ovary syndrome: comparison of 3 FSH-preparations.**
  Author(s): Department of Obstetrics and Gynecology, Klinikum Grosshadern, Ludwig Maximilians University Munich, Germany. Thomas.Strowitzki@gyn.med.uni-muenchen.de.
  Source: Strowitzki, T Seehaus, D Korell, M Hepp, H Exp-Clin-Endocrinol-Diabetes. 1998; 106(5): 435-9 0947-7349

- **Medication status and polycystic ovary syndrome in women with bipolar disorder: a preliminary report.**
  Author(s): Department of Psychiatry and Biobehavioral Sciences, University of California Los Angeles (UCLA), USA.
  Source: Rasgon, N L Altshuler, L L Gudeman, D Burt, V K Tanavoli, S Hendrick, V Korenman, S J-Clin-Psychiatry. 2000 March; 61(3): 173-8 0160-6689

- **Naltrexone effect on pulsatile GnRH therapy for ovulation induction in polycystic ovary syndrome: a pilot prospective study.**
  Author(s): Department of Obstetrics and Gynecology, Universita Cattolica del Sacro Cuore, Rome, Italy. alanzone@rm.unicatt.it
  Source: Fulghesu, A M Ciampelli, M Belosi, C Apa, R Guido, M Caruso, A Mancuso, S Lanzone, A J-Endocrinol-Invest. 2001 Jul-August; 24(7): 483-90 0391-4097

- **Obesity and the polycystic ovary syndrome.**
  Author(s): Endocrinology Unit, Department of Internal Medicine, S. Orsola-Malpighi Hospital, University Alma Mater Studiorum, Bologna, Italy.
  Source: Gambineri, A Pelusi, C Vicennati, V Pagotto, U Pasquali, R Int-J-Obes-Relat-Metab-Disord. 2002 July; 26(7): 883-96 0307-0565

- **Octreotide, a somatostatin analogue, alters ovarian sensitivity to gonadotrophin stimulation as measured by the follicle stimulating hormone threshold in polycystic ovary syndrome.**
  Author(s): Department of Obstetrics and Gynaecology, University Hospital Vrije Universiteit, Amsterdam, The Netherlands.
  Source: van der Meer, M de Boer, J A Hompes, P G Schoemaker, J Hum-Reprod. 1998 June; 13(6): 1465-9 0268-1161

- **Ovarian hyperstimulation after administration of triptorelin therapy to a patient with polycystic ovary syndrome.**
  Author(s): Department of Obstetrics and Gynecology, Catholic University of the Sacred Heart, Rome, Italy.
  Source: Campo, S Bezzi, I Garcea, N Fertil-Steril. 2000 June; 73(6): 1256-8 0015-0282

- **Ovarian morphology in long-term androgen-treated female to male transsexuals. A human model for the study of polycystic ovarian syndrome?**
  Author(s): Department of Obstetrics and Gynaecology, Dijkzigt University Hospital, Rotterdam, The Netherlands.
  Source: Pache, T D Chadha, S Gooren, L J Hop, W C Jaarsma, K W Dommerholt, H B Fauser, B C Histopathology. 1991 November; 19(5): 445-52 0309-0167

- **Ovarian stimulation with low-dose pure follicle-stimulating hormone in polycystic ovarian syndrome anovulatory patients: effect of long-term pretreatment with gonadotrophin-releasing hormone analogue.**
  Author(s): First Department of Obstetrics and Gynaecology, University of Milan, Italy.
  Source: Vegetti, W Testa, G Ragni, G Parazzini, F Crosignani, P G Gynecol-Obstet-Invest. 1998; 45(3): 186-9 0378-7346

- **Ovulation induction with urinary follicle stimulating hormone versus human menopausal gonadotropin for clomiphene-resistant polycystic ovary syndrome.**
  Author(s): Rm HSC-4F7, Department of Obstetrics and Gynaecology, McMaster University, 1200 Main St West, Hamilton, Ontario, Canada, L8N 3Z5. hughese@fhs.csu.mcmaster.ca
  Source: Hughes, E Collins, J Vandekerckhove, P Cochrane-Database-Syst-Revolume 2000; (2): CD000087 1469-493X

- **Pituitary and adrenal response to ovine corticotropin-releasing hormone in women with polycystic ovarian syndrome.**
  Author(s): Department of Internal Medicine, University of Catania, Italy.
  Source: Mongioi, A Macchi, M Vicari, E Fornito, M C Calogero, A E Riccioli, C Minacapilli, G Moncada, M L D'Agata, R J-Endocrinol-Invest. 1988 October; 11(9): 637-40 0391-4097

- **Polycystic ovarian syndrome in women with epilepsy: a review.**
  Author(s): Clinical Neurosciences Centre, Hope Hospital, Salford, Manchester, England, UK. susanduncan@compuserve.com
  Source: Duncan, S Epilepsia. 2001; 42 Suppl 3: 60-5 0013-9580

- **Polycystic ovaries, obesity and insulin resistance in women with epilepsy. A comparative study of carbamazepine and valproic acid in 105 women.**
  Author(s): Department of Neurology, University Hospital Innsbruck, Anichstrasse 35, Austria. gerhard.luef@uibk.ac.at
  Source: Luef, G Abraham, I Haslinger, M Trinka, E Seppi, K Unterberger, I Alge, A Windisch, J Lechleitner, M Bauer, G J-Neurol. 2002 July; 249(7): 835-41 0340-5354

- **Predictive value of serum androstenedione basal levels on the choice of gonadotropin or laparoscopic ovarian electrocautery as ovulation induction in clomiphene citrate-resistant patients with polycystic ovary syndrome.**
  Author(s): Department of Obstetrics and Gynecology, University of Bari, Italy.
  Source: Vicino, M Loverro, G Bettocchi, S Simonetti, S Mei, L Selvaggi, L Gynecol-Endocrinol. 2000 February; 14(1): 42-9 0951-3590

- **Pregnancy and delivery after cryopreservation of zygotes produced by in-vitro matured oocytes retrieved from a woman with polycystic ovarian syndrome.**
  Author(s): McGill Reproductive Center, Department of Obstetrics and Gynecology, McGill University, Montreal, Canada. rchian@tcartononline.com
  Source: Chian, R C Gulekli, B Buckett, W M Tan, S L Hum-Reprod. 2001 August; 16(8): 1700-2 0268-1161

- **Prospective randomized study of human chorionic gonadotrophin priming before immature oocyte retrieval from unstimulated women with polycystic ovarian syndrome.**
  Author(s): McGill Reproductive Center, Department of Obstetrics and Gynecology, Royal Victoria Hospital, McGill University, Montreal, Quebec, Canada H3A 1A1.
  Source: Chian, R C Buckett, W M Tulandi, T Tan, S L Hum-Reprod. 2000 January; 15(1): 165-70 0268-1161

- **Recombinant versus urinary follicle-stimulating hormone in the low-dose regimen in anovulatory patients with polycystic ovary syndrome: a safer and more effective treatment.**
  Author(s): Department of Obstetrics and Gynecology, Catholic University of Sacred Heart, Rome, Italy. fulg@tiscalinet.it
  Source: Fulghesu, A M Apa, R Belosi, C Ciampelli, M Selvaggi, L Jr Cucinelli, F Caruso, A Mancuso, S Lanzone, A Horm-Res. 2001; 55(5): 224-8 0301-0163

- **Selected aspects of polycystic ovarian disease.**
  Author(s): Department of Obstetrics and Gynecology, Baylor College of Medicine, Houston, Texas.
  Source: Goldzieher, J W Young, R L Endocrinol-Metab-Clin-North-Am. 1992 March; 21(1): 141-71 0889-8529

- **Should patients with polycystic ovarian syndrome be treated with metformin? A note of cautious optimism.**
  Author(s): Lis Maternity Hospital, Tel Aviv (Sourasky) Medical Centre, Tel Aviv 64239, Israel. homburg@netvision.net.il
  Source: Homburg, R Hum-Reprod. 2002 April; 17(4): 853-6 0268-1161

- **Sonographic monitoring of ovarian volume during LHRH analogue therapy in women with polycystic ovarian syndrome.**
  Author(s): Dept. of Obstetrics and Gynecology A, Meir General Hospital, Kfar-Sava, Israel.
  Source: Jaffe, R Abramowicz, J Eckstein, N Vagman, I Fejgin, M Ayalon, D J-Ultrasound-Med. 1988 April; 7(4): 203-6 0278-4297

- **Surgical or medical treatment of polycystic ovary syndrome: a cost-benefit analysis.**
  Author(s): Ovulation Induction Service, Department of Obstetrics and Gynaecology, Monash University, Prince Henry's Institute of Medical Research, Victoria, Australia.
  Source: Kovacs, G T Clarke, S Burger, H G Healy, D L Vollenhoven, B Gynecol-Endocrinol. 2002 February; 16(1): 53-5 0951-3590

- **The prevalence of polycystic ovaries in women with type 2 diabetes mellitus.**
  Author(s): Department of Medicine, University College London Medical School, The Middlesex Hospital, London, UK.
  Source: Conn, J J Jacobs, H S Conway, G S Clin-Endocrinol-(Oxf). 2000 January; 52(1): 81-6 0300-0664

- **The use of gonadotrophin-releasing hormone antagonists in polycystic ovarian disease.**
  Author(s): Service d'Endocrinologie, Hopital Saint Antoine, Paris, France.
  Source: Lubin, V Charbonnel, B Bouchard, P Baillieres-Clin-Obstet-Gynaecol. 1998 December; 12(4): 607-18 0950-3552

- **Therapeutic effects of metformin on insulin resistance and hyperandrogenism in polycystic ovary syndrome.**
  Author(s): University of Athens Medical School, First Department of Medicine, Laiko Athens General Hospital, Greece.
  Source: Diamanti Kandarakis, E Kouli, C Tsianateli, T Bergiele, A Eur-J-Endocrinol. 1998 March; 138(3): 269-74 0804-4643

- **Transvaginal ovarian drilling: a new surgical treatment for improving he clinical outcome of assisted reproductive technologies in patients with polycystic ovary syndrome.**
  Author(s): Reproductive Medicine Unit, Societa Italiana per gli Studi sulla Medicina della Riproduzione srl, Bologna, Italy. sismer@sismer.it
  Source: Ferraretti, A P Gianaroli, L Magli, M C Iammarrone, E Feliciani, E Fortini, D Fertil-Steril. 2001 October; 76(4): 812-6 0015-0282

- **Use of luteinizing hormone releasing hormone agonists in polycystic ovary syndrome.**
  Author(s): Department of Obstetrics and Gynecology, McGill University Royal Victoria Hospital, Montreal, Quebec, Canada.
  Source: Buckett, W M Tan, S L Baillieres-Clin-Obstet-Gynaecol. 1998 December; 12(4): 593-606 0950-3552

- **Utero-ovarian arterial blood flow and hormonal profile in patients with polycystic ovary syndrome.**
  Author(s): Department of Obstetrics and Gynaecology Ljubljana, University Medical Centre Ljubljana, Slovenia.
  Source: Vrtacnik Bokal, E Meden Vrtovec, H Hum-Reprod. 1998 April; 13(4): 815-21 0268-1161

- **Valproate, hyperandrogenism, and polycystic ovaries: a report of 3 cases.**
  Author(s): Department of Neurology, University of Oulu, FIN-90220 Oulu, Finland. jouko.isojarvi@oulu.fi.
  Source: Isojarvi, J I Tapanainen, J S Arch-Neurol. 2000 July; 57(7): 1064-8 0003-9942

- **Vitamin D and calcium dysregulation in the polycystic ovarian syndrome.**
  Author(s): Department of Medicine, St. Lukes-Roosevelt Hospital Center, Columbia University, College of Physicians & Surgeons, New York, NY 10019, USA.
  Source: Thys Jacobs, S Donovan, D Papadopoulos, A Sarrel, P Bilezikian, J P Steroids. 1999 June; 64(6): 430-5 0039-128X

Federal Resources on Nutrition

In addition to the IBIDS, the United States Department of Health and Human Services (HHS) and the United States Department of Agriculture (USDA) provide many sources of information on general nutrition and health. Recommended resources include:

- healthfinder®, HHS's gateway to health information, including diet and nutrition: http://www.healthfinder.gov/scripts/SearchContext.asp?topic=238&page=0

- The United States Department of Agriculture's Web site dedicated to nutrition information: **www.nutrition.gov**

- The Food and Drug Administration's Web site for federal food safety information: **www.foodsafety.gov**

- The National Action Plan on Overweight and Obesity sponsored by the United States Surgeon General: **http://www.surgeongeneral.gov/topics/obesity/**
- The Center for Food Safety and Applied Nutrition has an Internet site sponsored by the Food and Drug Administration and the Department of Health and Human Services: **http://vm.cfsan.fda.gov/**
- Center for Nutrition Policy and Promotion sponsored by the United States Department of Agriculture: **http://www.usda.gov/cnpp/**
- Food and Nutrition Information Center, National Agricultural Library sponsored by the United States Department of Agriculture: **http://www.nal.usda.gov/fnic/**
- Food and Nutrition Service sponsored by the United States Department of Agriculture: **http://www.fns.usda.gov/fns/**

Additional Web Resources

A number of additional Web sites offer encyclopedic information covering food and nutrition. The following is a representative sample:

- AOL: **http://search.aol.com/cat.adp?id=174&layer=&from=subcats**
- Family Village: **http://www.familyvillage.wisc.edu/med_nutrition.html**
- Google: **http://directory.google.com/Top/Health/Nutrition/**
- Healthnotes: **http://www.healthnotes.com/**
- Open Directory Project: **http://dmoz.org/Health/Nutrition/**
- Yahoo.com: **http://dir.yahoo.com/Health/Nutrition/**
- WebMD®Health: **http://my.webmd.com/nutrition**
- WholeHealthMD.com: **http://www.wholehealthmd.com/reflib/0,1529,00.html**

The following is a specific Web list relating to polycystic ovarian syndrome; please note that any particular subject below may indicate either a therapeutic use, or a contraindication (potential danger), and does not reflect an official recommendation:

- **Minerals**

    Calcium
    Source: Healthnotes, Inc.; www.healthnotes.com

CHAPTER 3. ALTERNATIVE MEDICINE AND POLYCYSTIC OVARIAN SYNDROME

Overview

In this chapter, we will begin by introducing you to official information sources on complementary and alternative medicine (CAM) relating to polycystic ovarian syndrome. At the conclusion of this chapter, we will provide additional sources.

National Center for Complementary and Alternative Medicine

The National Center for Complementary and Alternative Medicine (NCCAM) of the National Institutes of Health (http://nccam.nih.gov/) has created a link to the National Library of Medicine's databases to facilitate research for articles that specifically relate to polycystic ovarian syndrome and complementary medicine. To search the database, go to the following Web site: **http://www.nlm.nih.gov/nccam/camonpubmed.html**. Select "CAM on PubMed." Enter "polycystic ovarian syndrome" (or synonyms) into the search box. Click "Go." The following references provide information on particular aspects of complementary and alternative medicine that are related to polycystic ovarian syndrome:

- **Acupuncture normalizes dysfunction of hypothalamic-pituitary-ovarian axis.**
  Author(s): Chen BY.
  Source: Acupuncture & Electro-Therapeutics Research. 1997; 22(2): 97-108.
  http://www.ncbi.nlm.nih.gov:80/entrez/query.fcgi?cmd=Retrieve&db=PubMed&list_uids=9330669&dopt=Abstract

- **Case reports.**
  Author(s): Betts T.
  Source: Seizure : the Journal of the British Epilepsy Association. 2002 April; 11 Suppl A: 229-31; Quiz 232-4.
  http://www.ncbi.nlm.nih.gov:80/entrez/query.fcgi?cmd=Retrieve&db=PubMed&list_uids=12185761&dopt=Abstract

- **Clinical utility of adjuvant growth hormone in the treatment of patients with polycystic ovaries undergoing in vitro fertilization.**

Author(s): Artini PG, de Micheroux AA, Taponeco F, Cela V, D'Ambrogio G, Genazzani AR.
Source: Journal of Assisted Reproduction and Genetics. 1997 January; 14(1): 4-7. Review.
http://www.ncbi.nlm.nih.gov:80/entrez/query.fcgi?cmd=Retrieve&db=PubMed&list_uids=9013300&dopt=Abstract

- **Effect of a traditional herbal medicine (shakuyaku-kanzo-to) on testosterone secretion in patients with polycystic ovary syndrome detected by ultrasound.**
  Author(s): Takahashi K, Yoshino K, Shirai T, Nishigaki A, Araki Y, Kitao M.
  Source: Nippon Sanka Fujinka Gakkai Zasshi. 1988 June; 40(6): 789-92.
  http://www.ncbi.nlm.nih.gov:80/entrez/query.fcgi?cmd=Retrieve&db=PubMed&list_uids=3292675&dopt=Abstract

- **Effect of TJ-68 (shakuyaku-kanzo-to) on polycystic ovarian disease.**
  Author(s): Takahashi K, Kitao M.
  Source: Int J Fertil Menopausal Stud. 1994 March-April; 39(2): 69-76.
  http://www.ncbi.nlm.nih.gov:80/entrez/query.fcgi?cmd=Retrieve&db=PubMed&list_uids=8012442&dopt=Abstract

- **Effects of electro-acupuncture on anovulation in women with polycystic ovary syndrome.**
  Author(s): Stener-Victorin E, Waldenstrom U, Tagnfors U, Lundeberg T, Lindstedt G, Janson PO.
  Source: Acta Obstetricia Et Gynecologica Scandinavica. 2000 March; 79(3): 180-8.
  http://www.ncbi.nlm.nih.gov:80/entrez/query.fcgi?cmd=Retrieve&db=PubMed&list_uids=10716298&dopt=Abstract

- **Effects of electro-acupuncture on corticotropin-releasing factor in rats with experimentally-induced polycystic ovaries.**
  Author(s): Stener-Victorin E, Lundeberg T, Waldenstrom U, Bileviciute-Ljungar I, Janson PO.
  Source: Neuropeptides. 2001 October-December; 35(5-6): 227-31.
  http://www.ncbi.nlm.nih.gov:80/entrez/query.fcgi?cmd=Retrieve&db=PubMed&list_uids=12030806&dopt=Abstract

- **Effects of electro-acupuncture on nerve growth factor and ovarian morphology in rats with experimentally induced polycystic ovaries.**
  Author(s): Stener-Victorin E, Lundeberg T, Waldenstrom U, Manni L, Aloe L, Gunnarsson S, Janson PO.
  Source: Biology of Reproduction. 2000 November; 63(5): 1497-503.
  http://www.ncbi.nlm.nih.gov:80/entrez/query.fcgi?cmd=Retrieve&db=PubMed&list_uids=11058557&dopt=Abstract

- **Effects of unkei-to, an herbal medicine, on endocrine function and ovulation in women with high basal levels of luteinizing hormone secretion.**
  Author(s): Ushiroyama T, Ikeda A, Sakai M, Hosotani T, Suzuki Y, Tsubokura S, Ueki M.

Source: J Reprod Med. 2001 May; 46(5): 451-6.
http://www.ncbi.nlm.nih.gov:80/entrez/query.fcgi?cmd=Retrieve&db=PubMed&list_uids=11396371&dopt=Abstract

- **Frequency of a polymorphism in the regulatory region of the 17 alpha-hydroxylase-17,20-lyase (CYP17) gene in hyperandrogenic states.**
  Author(s): Techatraisak K, Conway GS, Rumsby G.
  Source: Clinical Endocrinology. 1997 February; 46(2): 131-4.
  http://www.ncbi.nlm.nih.gov:80/entrez/query.fcgi?cmd=Retrieve&db=PubMed&list_uids=9135692&dopt=Abstract

- **High incidence of preeclamptic toxemia in patients with polycystic ovarian disease.**
  Author(s): Diamant YZ, Rimon E, Evron S.
  Source: European Journal of Obstetrics, Gynecology, and Reproductive Biology. 1982 December; 14(3): 199-204.
  http://www.ncbi.nlm.nih.gov:80/entrez/query.fcgi?cmd=Retrieve&db=PubMed&list_uids=7160531&dopt=Abstract

- **In vivo and in vitro effects of gamma-linolenic acid and eicosapentaenoic acid on prostaglandin production and arachidonic acid uptake by human endometrium.**
  Author(s): Graham J, Franks S, Bonney RC.
  Source: Prostaglandins, Leukotrienes, and Essential Fatty Acids. 1994 June; 50(6): 321-9.
  http://www.ncbi.nlm.nih.gov:80/entrez/query.fcgi?cmd=Retrieve&db=PubMed&list_uids=7938084&dopt=Abstract

- **Induction of ovulation by Sairei-to for polycystic ovary syndrome patients.**
  Author(s): Sakai A, Kondo Z, Kamei K, Izumi S, Sumi K.
  Source: Endocrine Journal. 1999 February; 46(1): 217-20.
  http://www.ncbi.nlm.nih.gov:80/entrez/query.fcgi?cmd=Retrieve&db=PubMed&list_uids=10426590&dopt=Abstract

- **Induction of ovulation with traditional Chinese medicine.**
  Author(s): Ge QS, Zhang YW, Shen LZ.
  Source: J Tradit Chin Med. 1982 September; 2(3): 201-6. No Abstract Available.
  http://www.ncbi.nlm.nih.gov:80/entrez/query.fcgi?cmd=Retrieve&db=PubMed&list_uids=6765714&dopt=Abstract

- **Ovarian hyperstimulation syndrome after superovulation using GnRH agonists for IVF and related procedures.**
  Author(s): Rizk B, Smitz J.
  Source: Human Reproduction (Oxford, England). 1992 March; 7(3): 320-7. Review.
  http://www.ncbi.nlm.nih.gov:80/entrez/query.fcgi?cmd=Retrieve&db=PubMed&list_uids=1587936&dopt=Abstract

- **Polycystic ovary syndrome: clinical considerations.**
  Author(s): Marshall K.

Source: Alternative Medicine Review : a Journal of Clinical Therapeutic. 2001 June; 6(3): 272-92. Review.
http://www.ncbi.nlm.nih.gov:80/entrez/query.fcgi?cmd=Retrieve&db=PubMed&list_uids=11410072&dopt=Abstract

- **Pregnancies and deliveries after in vitro maturation culture followed by in vitro fertilization and embryo transfer without stimulation in women with polycystic ovary syndrome.**
  Author(s): Cha KY, Han SY, Chung HM, Choi DH, Lim JM, Lee WS, Ko JJ, Yoon TK.
  Source: Fertility and Sterility. 2000 May; 73(5): 978-83.
  http://www.ncbi.nlm.nih.gov:80/entrez/query.fcgi?cmd=Retrieve&db=PubMed&list_uids=10785224&dopt=Abstract

- **Self-selected women with polycystic ovary syndrome are reproductively and metabolically abnormal and undertreated.**
  Author(s): Legro RS, Urbanek M, Kunselman AR, Leiby BE, Dunaif A.
  Source: Fertility and Sterility. 2002 July; 78(1): 51-7.
  http://www.ncbi.nlm.nih.gov:80/entrez/query.fcgi?cmd=Retrieve&db=PubMed&list_uids=12095490&dopt=Abstract

- **The cytology of amenorrhoea.**
  Author(s): Wachtel E.
  Source: Acta Cytol. 1966 January-February; 10(1): 56-61. No Abstract Available.
  http://www.ncbi.nlm.nih.gov:80/entrez/query.fcgi?cmd=Retrieve&db=PubMed&list_uids=5220491&dopt=Abstract

- **The gonadotrophin surge in humans: its mechanism and role in ovulatory function--a review.**
  Author(s): Goh HH, Ratnam SS.
  Source: Ann Acad Med Singapore. 1990 July; 19(4): 524-9. Review.
  http://www.ncbi.nlm.nih.gov:80/entrez/query.fcgi?cmd=Retrieve&db=PubMed&list_uids=2221813&dopt=Abstract

- **'The thief of womanhood': women's experience of polycystic ovarian syndrome.**
  Author(s): Kitzinger C, Willmott J.
  Source: Social Science & Medicine (1982). 2002 February; 54(3): 349-61.
  http://www.ncbi.nlm.nih.gov:80/entrez/query.fcgi?cmd=Retrieve&db=PubMed&list_uids=11824912&dopt=Abstract

- **Treatment of polycystic ovary syndrome with Chinese drug longdan xiegan tang.**
  Author(s): Wang DZ, Wang ZQ, Shi LY.
  Source: J Tradit Chin Med. 1988 June; 8(2): 117-9. No Abstract Available.
  http://www.ncbi.nlm.nih.gov:80/entrez/query.fcgi?cmd=Retrieve&db=PubMed&list_uids=3412006&dopt=Abstract

- **Ultrasonographic guided ovarian stroma hydrocoagulation for ovarian stimulation in polycystic ovary syndrome.**
  Author(s): Ramzy AM, Al-Inany H, Aboulfoutouh I, Sataar M, Idrees OA, Shehata MH.

Source: Acta Obstetricia Et Gynecologica Scandinavica. 2001 November; 80(11): 1046-50.
http://www.ncbi.nlm.nih.gov:80/entrez/query.fcgi?cmd=Retrieve&db=PubMed&list_uids=11703206&dopt=Abstract

- **Urinary retention in women.**
  Author(s): Fowler CJ.
  Source: Bju International. 2003 April; 91(6): 463-4.
  http://www.ncbi.nlm.nih.gov:80/entrez/query.fcgi?cmd=Retrieve&db=PubMed&list_uids=12656891&dopt=Abstract

- **Was Robert Whytt (1714--1766) right? Remarks on the retirement of John C. Nemiah as psychiatrist-in-chief; Beth Israel Hospital.**
  Author(s): Weiner H.
  Source: Psychotherapy and Psychosomatics. 1986; 45(1): 5-13.
  http://www.ncbi.nlm.nih.gov:80/entrez/query.fcgi?cmd=Retrieve&db=PubMed&list_uids=3532160&dopt=Abstract

Additional Web Resources

A number of additional Web sites offer encyclopedic information covering CAM and related topics. The following is a representative sample:

- Alternative Medicine Foundation, Inc.: **http://www.herbmed.org/**
- AOL: **http://search.aol.com/cat.adp?id=169&layer=&from=subcats**
- Chinese Medicine: **http://www.newcenturynutrition.com/**
- drkoop.com®: **http://www.drkoop.com/InteractiveMedicine/IndexC.html**
- Family Village: **http://www.familyvillage.wisc.edu/med_altn.htm**
- Google: **http://directory.google.com/Top/Health/Alternative/**
- Healthnotes: **http://www.healthnotes.com/**
- MedWebPlus: **http://medwebplus.com/subject/Alternative_and_Complementary_Medicine**
- Open Directory Project: **http://dmoz.org/Health/Alternative/**
- HealthGate: **http://www.tnp.com/**
- WebMD®Health: **http://my.webmd.com/drugs_and_herbs**
- WholeHealthMD.com: **http://www.wholehealthmd.com/reflib/0,1529,00.html**
- Yahoo.com: **http://dir.yahoo.com/Health/Alternative_Medicine/**

The following is a specific Web list relating to polycystic ovarian syndrome; please note that any particular subject below may indicate either a therapeutic use, or a contraindication (potential danger), and does not reflect an official recommendation:

- **General Overview**

    Amenorrhea
    Source: Healthnotes, Inc.; www.healthnotes.com

    Diabetes Mellitus
    Source: Integrative Medicine Communications; www.drkoop.com

    High Cholesterol
    Source: Integrative Medicine Communications; www.drkoop.com

    Hirsuitism
    Source: Integrative Medicine Communications; www.drkoop.com

    Hypercholesterolemia
    Source: Integrative Medicine Communications; www.drkoop.com

    Obesity
    Source: Integrative Medicine Communications; www.drkoop.com

- **Alternative Therapy**

    Acupuncture
    Source: Integrative Medicine Communications; www.drkoop.com

- **Herbs and Supplements**

    Glycyrrhiza
    Alternative names: Licorice; Glycyrrhiza glabra L.
    Source: Alternative Medicine Foundation, Inc.; www.amfoundation.org

General References

A good place to find general background information on CAM is the National Library of Medicine. It has prepared within the MEDLINEplus system an information topic page dedicated to complementary and alternative medicine. To access this page, go to the MEDLINEplus site at **http://www.nlm.nih.gov/medlineplus/alternativemedicine.html**. This Web site provides a general overview of various topics and can lead to a number of general sources.

CHAPTER 4. DISSERTATIONS ON POLYCYSTIC OVARIAN SYNDROME

Overview

In this chapter, we will give you a bibliography on recent dissertations relating to polycystic ovarian syndrome. We will also provide you with information on how to use the Internet to stay current on dissertations. **IMPORTANT NOTE:** When following the search strategy described below, you may discover non-medical dissertations that use the generic term "polycystic ovarian syndrome" (or a synonym) in their titles. To accurately reflect the results that you might find while conducting research on polycystic ovarian syndrome, we have not necessarily excluded non-medical dissertations in this bibliography.

Dissertations on Polycystic Ovarian Syndrome

ProQuest Digital Dissertations, the largest archive of academic dissertations available, is located at the following Web address: **http://wwwlib.umi.com/dissertations**. From this archive, we have compiled the following list covering dissertations devoted to polycystic ovarian syndrome. You will see that the information provided includes the dissertation's title, its author, and the institution with which the author is associated. The following covers recent dissertations found when using this search procedure:

- **The Influence of Hyperandrogenism, Obesity and Infertility on the Psychosocial Health and Well-Being of Women with Polycystic Ovary Syndrome** by McCook, Judy Griffin; PhD from University of Michigan, 2002, 150 pages
  http://wwwlib.umi.com/dissertations/fullcit/3042131

- **The Prenatally Androgenized Female Rhesus Monkey As a Model for Polycystic Ovary Syndrome** by Eisner, Joel Robert; PhD from The University of Wisconsin - Madison, 2002, 166 pages
  http://wwwlib.umi.com/dissertations/fullcit/3049500

- **Transcriptional Regulation of the 17alpha-hydroxylase Gene in Normal and Polycystic Ovary Syndrome Ovarian Theca Cells** by Wickenheisser, Jessica Katherine; PhD from The Pennsylvania State University, 2002, 180 pages
  http://wwwlib.umi.com/dissertations/fullcit/3077599

Keeping Current

Ask the medical librarian at your library if it has full and unlimited access to the *ProQuest Digital Dissertations* database. From the library, you should be able to do more complete searches via **http://wwwlib.umi.com/dissertations**.

Chapter 5. Clinical Trials and Polycystic Ovarian Syndrome

Overview

In this chapter, we will show you how to keep informed of the latest clinical trials concerning polycystic ovarian syndrome.

Recent Trials on Polycystic Ovarian Syndrome

The following is a list of recent trials dedicated to polycystic ovarian syndrome.[8] Further information on a trial is available at the Web site indicated.

- **Randomized Study of Decreased Hyperinsulinemia on the Ovulatory Response to Clomiphene Citrate in Women With Polycystic Ovary Syndrome**

    Condition(s): Polycystic Ovary Syndrome; Hyperinsulinism

    Study Status: This study is currently recruiting patients.

    Sponsor(s): National Center for Research Resources (NCRR); University of Virginia

    Purpose - Excerpt: Objectives: I. Determine whether reduction of serum insulin levels by metformin increases ovulatory response to clomiphene citrate in women with **polycystic ovary syndrome.**

    Study Type: Interventional

    Contact(s): see Web site below

    Web Site: http://clinicaltrials.gov/ct/show/NCT00005104

- **Treatment of Infertility in Women With Polycystic Ovary Syndrome**

    Condition(s): Polycystic Ovary Syndrome; Infertility; Pregnancy

    Study Status: This study is currently recruiting patients.

    Sponsor(s): National Institute of Child Health and Human Development (NICHD)

---

[8] These are listed at **www.ClinicalTrials.gov**.

Purpose - Excerpt: Polycystic Ovary Syndrome (PCOS) is a common endocrine disorder affecting up to 10% of women. The primary symptoms of PCOS are menstrual irregularities, increased body and facial hair, acne, and infertility. This study will test a combination of medications in women with PCOS to determine which works best to overcome infertility.

Phase(s): Phase III

Study Type: Interventional

Contact(s): see Web site below

Web Site: http://clinicaltrials.gov/ct/show/NCT00068861

- **Androgens and Subclinical Atherosclerosis in Young Women - Ancillary to CARDIA**

    Condition(s): Cardiovascular Diseases; Coronary Arteriosclerosis; Heart Diseases; Polycystic Ovary Syndrome

    Study Status: This study is no longer recruiting patients.

    Sponsor(s): National Heart, Lung, and Blood Institute (NHLBI)

    Purpose - Excerpt: To examine whether serum androgens, measured earlier in life, and variation in genes related to androgen synthesis, metabolism, and signaling are associated with early-onset subclinical coronary atherosclerosis in young adult women from the community.

    Study Type: Observational

    Contact(s): see Web site below

    Web Site: http://clinicaltrials.gov/ct/show/NCT00037245

- **Risk of Coronary Heart Disease in Women with Polycystic Ovary Syndrome**

    Condition(s): Atherosclerosis; Cardiovascular Diseases; Heart Diseases; Carotid Artery Diseases; Coronary Disease; Polycystic Ovary Syndrome

    Study Status: This study is no longer recruiting patients.

    Sponsor(s): National Heart, Lung, and Blood Institute (NHLBI)

    Purpose - Excerpt: To investigate whether women with **Polycystic Ovary syndrome** (PCOS) have evidence of an increased prevalence rate of subclinical atherosclerosis as measured by the presence of plaque, increased intima-medial carotid artery wall thickness and lower brachial artery flow mediated vasodilation.

    Study Type: Observational

    Contact(s): see Web site below

    Web Site: http://clinicaltrials.gov/ct/show/NCT00005459

- **Phase II Study of the Effect of Leuprolide Acetate and Spironolactone on Insulin Resistance in Hyperandrogenic Women with Polycystic Ovarian Disease or Hyperandrogenism Insulin Resistance Acanthosis Nigricans Syndrome**

    Condition(s): Acanthosis Nigricans; Polycystic Ovary Syndrome

    Study Status: This study is completed.

    Sponsor(s): National Center for Research Resources (NCRR); Baylor College of Medicine

Purpose - Excerpt: Objectives: I. Evaluate insulin resistance in thin and obese hyperandrogenic women with **polycystic ovarian disease** or hyperandrogenism insulin resistance acanthosis nigricans syndrome and in thin and obese controls, using an estimation of tissue sensitivity to insulin. II. Evaluate the effect of androgen suppression with leuprolide acetate and spironolactone on insulin secretion and resistance.

Phase(s): Phase II

Study Type: Interventional

Contact(s): see Web site below

Web Site: http://clinicaltrials.gov/ct/show/NCT00004311

- **Randomized Study of the Effect of Decreased Hyperinsulinemia on the Ovulatory Response to Clomiphene Citrate in Obese Women With Polycystic Ovary Syndrome**

  Condition(s): Hyperinsulinism; Polycystic Ovary Syndrome

  Study Status: This study is completed.

  Sponsor(s): National Center for Research Resources (NCRR); University of Virginia

  Purpose - Excerpt: Objectives: I. Determine whether reduction of serum insulin levels by metformin increases ovulatory response to clomiphene or spontaneous ovulation in obese women with **polycystic ovary syndrome.**

  Study Type: Interventional

  Contact(s): see Web site below

  Web Site: http://clinicaltrials.gov/ct/show/NCT00005654

Keeping Current on Clinical Trials

The U.S. National Institutes of Health, through the National Library of Medicine, has developed ClinicalTrials.gov to provide current information about clinical research across the broadest number of diseases and conditions.

The site was launched in February 2000 and currently contains approximately 5,700 clinical studies in over 59,000 locations worldwide, with most studies being conducted in the United States. ClinicalTrials.gov receives about 2 million hits per month and hosts approximately 5,400 visitors daily. To access this database, simply go to the Web site at **http://www.clinicaltrials.gov/** and search by "polycystic ovarian syndrome" (or synonyms).

While ClinicalTrials.gov is the most comprehensive listing of NIH-supported clinical trials available, not all trials are in the database. The database is updated regularly, so clinical trials are continually being added. The following is a list of specialty databases affiliated with the National Institutes of Health that offer additional information on trials:

- For clinical studies at the Warren Grant Magnuson Clinical Center located in Bethesda, Maryland, visit their Web site: **http://clinicalstudies.info.nih.gov/**

- For clinical studies conducted at the Bayview Campus in Baltimore, Maryland, visit their Web site: **http://www.jhbmc.jhu.edu/studies/index.html**

- For cancer trials, visit the National Cancer Institute: **http://cancertrials.nci.nih.gov/**

- For eye-related trials, visit and search the Web page of the National Eye Institute: **http://www.nei.nih.gov/neitrials/index.htm**
- For heart, lung and blood trials, visit the Web page of the National Heart, Lung and Blood Institute: **http://www.nhlbi.nih.gov/studies/index.htm**
- For trials on aging, visit and search the Web site of the National Institute on Aging: **http://www.grc.nia.nih.gov/studies/index.htm**
- For rare diseases, visit and search the Web site sponsored by the Office of Rare Diseases: **http://ord.aspensys.com/asp/resources/rsch_trials.asp**
- For alcoholism, visit the National Institute on Alcohol Abuse and Alcoholism: **http://www.niaaa.nih.gov/intramural/Web_dicbr_hp/particip.htm**
- For trials on infectious, immune, and allergic diseases, visit the site of the National Institute of Allergy and Infectious Diseases: **http://www.niaid.nih.gov/clintrials/**
- For trials on arthritis, musculoskeletal and skin diseases, visit newly revised site of the National Institute of Arthritis and Musculoskeletal and Skin Diseases of the National Institutes of Health: **http://www.niams.nih.gov/hi/studies/index.htm**
- For hearing-related trials, visit the National Institute on Deafness and Other Communication Disorders: **http://www.nidcd.nih.gov/health/clinical/index.htm**
- For trials on diseases of the digestive system and kidneys, and diabetes, visit the National Institute of Diabetes and Digestive and Kidney Diseases: **http://www.niddk.nih.gov/patient/patient.htm**
- For drug abuse trials, visit and search the Web site sponsored by the National Institute on Drug Abuse: **http://www.nida.nih.gov/CTN/Index.htm**
- For trials on mental disorders, visit and search the Web site of the National Institute of Mental Health: **http://www.nimh.nih.gov/studies/index.cfm**
- For trials on neurological disorders and stroke, visit and search the Web site sponsored by the National Institute of Neurological Disorders and Stroke of the NIH: **http://www.ninds.nih.gov/funding/funding_opportunities.htm#Clinical_Trials**

CHAPTER 6. PATENTS ON POLYCYSTIC OVARIAN SYNDROME

Overview

Patents can be physical innovations (e.g. chemicals, pharmaceuticals, medical equipment) or processes (e.g. treatments or diagnostic procedures). The United States Patent and Trademark Office defines a patent as a grant of a property right to the inventor, issued by the Patent and Trademark Office.[9] Patents, therefore, are intellectual property. For the United States, the term of a new patent is 20 years from the date when the patent application was filed. If the inventor wishes to receive economic benefits, it is likely that the invention will become commercially available within 20 years of the initial filing. It is important to understand, therefore, that an inventor's patent does not indicate that a product or service is or will be commercially available. The patent implies only that the inventor has "the right to exclude others from making, using, offering for sale, or selling" the invention in the United States. While this relates to U.S. patents, similar rules govern foreign patents.

In this chapter, we show you how to locate information on patents and their inventors. If you find a patent that is particularly interesting to you, contact the inventor or the assignee for further information. **IMPORTANT NOTE:** When following the search strategy described below, you may discover non-medical patents that use the generic term "polycystic ovarian syndrome" (or a synonym) in their titles. To accurately reflect the results that you might find while conducting research on polycystic ovarian syndrome, we have not necessarily excluded non-medical patents in this bibliography.

Patents on Polycystic Ovarian Syndrome

By performing a patent search focusing on polycystic ovarian syndrome, you can obtain information such as the title of the invention, the names of the inventor(s), the assignee(s) or the company that owns or controls the patent, a short abstract that summarizes the patent, and a few excerpts from the description of the patent. The abstract of a patent tends to be more technical in nature, while the description is often written for the public. Full patent

---

[9] Adapted from the United States Patent and Trademark Office: http://www.uspto.gov/web/offices/pac/doc/general/whatis.htm.

descriptions contain much more information than is presented here (e.g. claims, references, figures, diagrams, etc.). We will tell you how to obtain this information later in the chapter. The following is an example of the type of information that you can expect to obtain from a patent search on polycystic ovarian syndrome:

- **Method of treating polycystic ovarian syndrome**

    Inventor(s): Thys-Jacobs; Susan (Larchmont, NY)

    Assignee(s): The Trustees of Columbia University in the City of New York (New York, NY)

    Patent Number: 6,034,075

    Date filed: March 19, 1998

    Abstract: The present invention is directed to a method of treating **polycystic ovarian syndrome** (PCO) with calcium alone, with vitamin D alone, or with the combination calcium and vitamin D. This invention further provides a method of treating infertility in a woman which comprises administering to the subject an amount of calcium or a derivative thereof effective to treat the infertility. The present invention is also directed to a method of treating irregular menses (oligo/amenorrhea), acne, or hirsutism, insulin resistance, or infertility which comprises administering a combination of calcium or a derivative thereof and vitamin D or a derivative thereof in an amount effective to treat irregular menses (oligo/amenorrhea), acne, or hirsutism, insulin resistance, or infertility. This invention also provides a method of preventing **polycystic ovarian syndrome** which comprises administering to the subject a combination of vitamin D or a derivative thereof and calcium or a derivative thereof in an amount effective to prevent the onset of **polycystic ovarian syndrome.**

    Excerpt(s): Throughout this application, various publications are referenced by author and date. Full citations for these publications may be found listed alphabetically at the end of the specification immediately before the claims. The disclosures of these publications in their entireties are hereby incorporated by reference into this application in order to more fully describe the state of the art as known to those skilled therein. In 1935, Stein and Leventhal recognized the association of enlarged **polycystic ovaries** with amenorrhea, hirsutism and infertility. (Stein and Leventhal, 1935) Since then, the increased ovarian androgen production, hyperandrogenemia and menstrual irregularity have come to be known as **polycystic ovary syndrome.** (Rosenfeld, et al. 1972) **Polycystic ovarian syndrome** (PCO) has been described as one of the most common female endocrine disorders. Its incidence has been estimated to be about 5% in both adolescent and adult populations. (Declercq and van de Calseyde, 1977) It is characterized by hyperandrogenic chronic anovulation (increased androgen concentrations and cessation of ovulatory cycles), and clinically presents in the prepubertal period with any of the following: irregular menses, amenorrhea, dysfunctional uterine bleeding and hirsutism. (Frank, 1995) It is the most frequent cause of anovulation with approximately 55% of patients presenting with amenorrhea (absence of menses) and 70% with hirsutism. The syndrome comprises a spectrum of ovarian histological and morphological findings, ovarian steroid, gonadotropin and metabolic abnormalities. In recent years, PCO has been associated with a characteristic metabolic disturbance, insulin resistance and hyperinsulinemia. (Dunaif, et al., 1989) The hyperinsulinemia in PCO is not seen in all women but is more prevalent in obese young women. Evidence suggests that disordered insulin metabolism may precipitate increased androgen levels, while suppression of insulin levels with diazoxide or metformin can cause resumption of menses. Insulin stimulates androgen secretion in ovarian stroma in vitro and may act on the ovary via insulin growth factor receptors. (Barbieri, et al., 1986; Adashi, et al., 1985) The cellular mechanism underlying insulin resistance may reflect reduced binding of insulin to its receptor or a decreased expression of the insulin dependent glucose transporter protein GLT-4. (Jialal, et al.1987;Rosenbaum, et al., 1993) Treatment of PCO has traditionally been directed toward interrupting the self-perpetuating cycle of hormonal events. This has been done either with the use of surgery as in wedge resection of the ovary or through medical interventions by lowering LH levels (oral contraceptives and LHRH analogues). Other approaches have included enhancement of FSH secretion with clomiphene, human menopausal gonadotrophin or pulsatile LHRH therapy.

Web site: http://www.delphion.com/details?pn=US06034075__

- **Method of treating psychological and metabolic disorders using IGF or IGF/IGFBP-3**

  Inventor(s): Mascarenhas; Desmond (Los Altos Hills, CA)

  Assignee(s): Celtrix Pharmaceuticals, Inc. (Glen Allen, VA)

  Patent Number: 6,514,937

  Date filed: July 27, 1998

  Abstract: Methods are provided for treating or alleviating the symptoms of subjects with psychological disorders, metabolic disorders, chronic stress-related disorders, sleep disorders, conditions associated with sexual senescence, aging, or premature aging by treating such subjects with IGF or mutant IGF either alone or complexed with IGFBP-3. Methods for increasing the levels of DHEA or DHEAS and treating or alleviating the symptoms of subjects with disorders characterized by low levels of DHEA or DHEAS by administering effective amounts of IGF or mutant IGF alone or complexed with IGFBP-3 are also provided. Methods for increasing the level of T4 and treating or alleviating the symptoms of subjects with disorders characterized by low levels of T3 or T4 by administering effective amounts of IGF or mutant IGF alone or complexed with IGFBP-3 are additionally provided. Also provided are methods for the treatment of **polycystic ovarian syndrome** (PCOS) by long term administration of IGF/IGFBP-3 complex.

  Excerpt(s): The invention relates generally to the field of treating psychological and metabolic disorders, and relates particularly to the treatment of these disorders by administering insulin-like growth factor (IGF) alone or complexed with insulin-like growth factor binding protein-3 (IGFBP-3). Dehydroepiandrosterone (DHEA) and its sulfated form, dehydroepiandrosterone-sulfate (DHEAS) are the principal circulating steroids in humans. These two steroids are synthesized in the adrenal cortex and are normally found at about a 1:1000 molar ratio in serum. DHEAS is thought to be the storage form of DHEA, and can be converted to DHEA by the action of a sulfatase. DHEA can serve as a substrate for the production of androgenic steroids, both in the steroidogenic organs (adrenal glands, gonads and placenta) and in peripheral tissues, such as the skin, liver and brain. Administration of DHEA has been reported to increase serum levels of IGF-I (U.S. Pat. No. 5,407,927; Morales et al. (1994) J. Clin. Endocrinol. Metab. 78(6):1360-1367) and to increase the sense of well-being, but not the libido, of subjects receiving DHEA. However, these reports do not establish any linkage between the elevation of IGF-I levels and an improved sense of well-being.

  Web site: http://www.delphion.com/details?pn=US06514937__

- **Use of thiazolidinedione derivatives in the treatment of polycystic ovary syndrome, gestational diabetes and disease states at risk for progressing to noninsulin-dependent diabetes mellitus**

  Inventor(s): Antonucci; Tammy (Thousand Oaks, CA), Lockwood; Dean (Ann Arbor, MI), Norris; Rebecca (Kewadin, MI)

  Assignee(s): Warner-Lambert Company (Morris Plains, NJ)

  Patent Number: 5,874,454

  Date filed: May 15, 1997

  Abstract: Novel methods of using thiazolidinone derivatives and related antihyperglycemic agents to treat populations at risk for developing noninsulin-dependent diabetes mellitus (NIDDM) and complications arising therefrom are disclosed In one embodiment, the compounds of the invention are used to treat **polycystic ovary syndrome** in order to prevent or delay the onset of noninsulin-dependent diabetes mellitus. In another embodiment, the compounds of the invention are used to treat gestational diabetes in order to prevent or delay the onset of noninsulin-dependent diabetes mellitus.

  Excerpt(s): The present invention pertains to a number of compounds which can be used to treat certain disease states in order to prevent or delay the onset of noninsulin-dependent diabetes mellitus (NIDDM). More specifically, the present invention involves in one embodiment administering to a patient certain known thiazolidinedione derivatives and related antihyperglycemic agents which treat disease states such as polycystic ovary and gestational diabetes syndrome which are at increased risk in the development of NIDDM, thus preventing or delaying the onset of NIDDM or complications resulting therefrom. Diabetes is one of the most prevalent chronic disorders worldwide with significant personal and financial costs for patients and their families, as well as for society. Different types of diabetes exist with distinct etiologies and pathogeneses. For example, diabetes mellitus is a disorder of carbohydrate metabolism, characterized by hyperglycemia and glycosuria and resulting from inadequate production or utilization of insulin. Reports indicate that insulin secretion is often enhanced early-on, presumably as compensation for the insulin resistance. People who actually develop NIDDM appear to do so because their B-cells eventually fail to maintain sufficient insulin secretion to compensate for the insulin resistance. Mechanisms responsible for the Bcell failure have not been identified, but may be related to the chronic demands placed on the Bcells by peripheral insulin resistance and/or to the effects of hyperglycemia to impair B-cell function. The B-cell failure could also occur as an independent, inherent defect in "pre-diabetic" individuals.

  Web site: http://www.delphion.com/details?pn=US05874454__

Patent Applications on Polycystic Ovarian Syndrome

As of December 2000, U.S. patent applications are open to public viewing.[10] Applications are patent requests which have yet to be granted. (The process to achieve a patent can take several years.) The following patent applications have been filed since December 2000 relating to polycystic ovarian syndrome:

---

[10] This has been a common practice outside the United States prior to December 2000.

- **Compositions and methods for contraception and for treatment of benign gynecological disorders**

    Inventor(s): Daniels, John R.; (Pacific Palisades, CA), Pike, Malcolm Cecil; (Long Beach, CA), Spicer, Darcy V.; (Pasadena, CA)

    Correspondence: Christie, Parker & Hale, Llp; 350 West Colorado Boulevard; Suite 500; Pasadena; CA; 91105; US

    Patent Application Number: 20010016578

    Date filed: May 1, 2001

    Abstract: Compositions and methods for use in preventing conception or treating benign gynecological disorders, wherein an effective amount of an antiprogestational agent [e.g., progesterone (progestin, progestogen, gestagen) antagonist or progesterone synthesis inhibitor] administered over a first period of time is combined with an effective amount of a progestogen for a second period of time. The antiprogestational agent is selected from single agents or mixtures thereof. The progestogen is selected from single agents or mixtures of natural or synthetic progestogens. The formulations are effective as contraceptive agents and for treatment of benign gynecological disorders including uterine fibroids, premenstrual syndrome, dysfunctional uterine bleeding, **polycystic ovarian syndrome** and endometriosis.

    Excerpt(s): This invention relates to compositions and methods useful for contraception and for treatment of benign gynecological disorders in mammals, especially human females. More particularly, the present invention is directed to contraceptive methods and methods of treating benign gynecological disorders and preparations for use therein which are effective for reducing exposure to progestational agents. The first progestogen antagonist synthesized and tested was RU 486 [RU 38486; 17-hydroxy-11-(4-dimethylaminophenyl)-17-(prop-1-ynyl)estra-4,- 9-dien-3-one; beta-[(4-N,N-dimethylaminno)-phenyl]-17.beta.-hydroxy-17.alp- ha.-propynyl-4,9(10)-oestradiene-3-one; mefepristone]. Mefepristone has high affinity for the progesterone receptor, with predominantly antiprogestational effects. Mefepristone is known to have growth-inhibitory effects in breast cancer cells in in vitro and in vivo preclinical studies and in human clinical trials [Klijn, J. G. M. et al., Cancer Research 49:2851-2856 (1989)]. Other antiprogestational agents have been synthesized and tested including ZK 98.299 (onapristone) and ZK 112.993, which also have antitumor efficacy [Michna, H. et al., J. Sieroid Biochem. Molec. Biol. 43:203-210 (1992)]. Mefepristone is known to be useful as a medical abortifacient (because of its antiprogestational activities) and as a postcoital contraceptive. Mefepristone has been evaluated as a potential contraceptive agent using several schedules. A single dose of mefepristone late in the menstrual cycle may be a useful contraceptive approach [Nieman, L. K. et al., N. Engl. J. Med. 316:187-191 (1987)].

    Web site: http://appft1.uspto.gov/netahtml/PTO/search-bool.html

- **Genes regulated by peroxisome proliferator-activated receptor gamma agonist**

    Inventor(s): Schebye, Xiao Min; (San Carlos, CA)

    Correspondence: Incyte Genomics, INC.; 3160 Porter Drive; Palo Alto; CA; 94304; US

    Patent Application Number: 20030096272

    Date filed: July 29, 2002

Abstract: The present invention relates to a combination comprising a plurality of cDNAs which are differentially expressed in response to peroxisome proliferator-activated receptor gamma (PPAR.gamma.) agonist and which may be used entirely or in part to diagnose, to stage, to treat, or to monitor the progression or treatment of disorders such as diabetes mellitus, obesity, hypertension, atherosclerosis, **polycystic ovarian syndrome,** and cancers of the breast, prostate, or colon.

Excerpt(s): This application claims benefit of provisional application Serial No. 60/308,868, filed Jul. 30, 2001. Thiazolidinediones (TZDs) act as agonists for the peroxisome-proliferator-activated receptor gamma (PPAR.gamma.), a member of the nuclear hormone receptor superfamily. TZDs reduce hyperglycemia, hyperinsulinemia, and hypertension, in part by promoting glucose metabolism and inhibiting gluconeogenesis. Roles for PPAR.gamma. and its agonists have been demonstrated in a wide range of pathological conditions including diabetes, obesity, hypertension, atherosclerosis, **polycystic ovarian syndrome,** and cancers such as breast, prostate, and colon cancer and liposarcoma.

Web site: http://appft1.uspto.gov/netahtml/PTO/search-bool.html

- **Methods and compositions for the benefit of those suffering from polycystic ovary syndrome with chromium complexes**

    Inventor(s): Katz, David P.; (Dobbs Ferry, NY)

    Correspondence: Knobbe Martens Olson & Bear Llp; 620 Newport Center Drive; Sixteenth Floor; Newport Beach; CA; 92660; US

    Patent Application Number: 20020086065

    Date filed: October 25, 2001

    Abstract: Compositions comprising chromium complexes such as chromium picolinate or chromium nicotinate are administered to a subject presenting with **Polycystic Ovary Syndrome.** The compositions may further comprise at least one of a chelating agent, cyclooxygenase inhibitor, a mucolytic, and/or a salicin-containing herb.

    Excerpt(s): This application claims priority to Provisional Application No. 60/244,791 entitled METHODS AND COMPOSITIONS FOR THE BENEFIT OF THOSE SUFFERING FROM **POLYCYSTIC OVARY SYNDROME** WITH CHROMIUM COMPLEXES filed on Oct. 31, 2000. The subject matter of the aforementioned application is hereby incorporated by reference. The disclosed invention relates to compositions comprising chromium complexes and uses of these compositions in treating **Polycystic Ovary Syndrome** (PCOS). Polycystic Ovary Syndrome (PCOS) or **Stein-Leventhal Syndrome** affects an estimated 5% to 10% of women. The condition is characterized by 1) irregular or absent menses, 2) numerous cysts on the ovaries, 3) high blood pressure, 4) acne, 5) elevated insulin levels, insulin resistance, or type II diabetes, 6) infertility, 7) excess hair on the face or body, 8) male-pattern baldness, 9) abdominal obesity, and 10) abnormal lipid profiles.

    Web site: http://appft1.uspto.gov/netahtml/PTO/search-bool.html

- **Use of D-chiro-inositol in the treatment of conditions associated with hypothalamic gene expression**

    Inventor(s): Allan, Geoffrey; (Richmond, VA), Mobbs, Charles V.; (New York, NY)

    Correspondence: Sterne, Kessler, Goldstein & Fox Pllc; 1100 New York Avenue, N.W., Suite 600; Washington; DC; 20005-3934; US

    Patent Application Number: 20020032177

    Date filed: April 30, 2001

    Excerpt(s): This application claims benefit under 35 U.S.C.sctn. 119(e) of U.S. Provisional Application No. 60/200,471, filed Apr. 28, 2000. The present invention relates to the use of D-chiro-inositol (DCI) as a regulator of hypothalamic gene expression and, more particularly, to the use of DCI and derivatives and metabolites thereof to treat neuroendocrine impairments such as obesity, **polycystic ovarian syndrome** (PCOS), impaired regulation of hormones during aging and to correct such neuroendocrine impairments and associated functions. Obesity, especially upper body obesity, is a common and very serious public health problem in the United States and throughout the world. According to recent statistics, more than 25% of the United States population and 27% of the Canadian population are overweight (Kuczmarski Amer. J. Clin. Nutr. 55:495S502S (1992); Reeder et. al., Can. Med. Ass. J. 23: 226-233 (1992)). Upper body obesity is the strongest risk factor known for type II diabetes mellitus, and is a strong risk factor for cardiovascular disease and cancer as well. Recent estimates for the medical cost of obesity are $150,000,000,000 world wide. The problem has become serious enough that the surgeon general has begun an initiative to combat the ever increasing obesity rampant in American society.

    Web site: http://appft1.uspto.gov/netahtml/PTO/search-bool.html

Keeping Current

In order to stay informed about patents and patent applications dealing with polycystic ovarian syndrome, you can access the U.S. Patent Office archive via the Internet at the following Web address: **http://www.uspto.gov/patft/index.html**. You will see two broad options: (1) Issued Patent, and (2) Published Applications. To see a list of issued patents, perform the following steps: Under "Issued Patents," click "Quick Search." Then, type "polycystic ovarian syndrome" (or synonyms) into the "Term 1" box. After clicking on the search button, scroll down to see the various patents which have been granted to date on polycystic ovarian syndrome.

You can also use this procedure to view pending patent applications concerning polycystic ovarian syndrome. Simply go back to **http://www.uspto.gov/patft/index.html**. Select "Quick Search" under "Published Applications." Then proceed with the steps listed above.

CHAPTER 7. BOOKS ON POLYCYSTIC OVARIAN SYNDROME

Overview

This chapter provides bibliographic book references relating to polycystic ovarian syndrome. In addition to online booksellers such as www.amazon.com and www.bn.com, excellent sources for book titles on polycystic ovarian syndrome include the Combined Health Information Database and the National Library of Medicine. Your local medical library also may have these titles available for loan.

Book Summaries: Online Booksellers

Commercial Internet-based booksellers, such as Amazon.com and Barnes&Noble.com, offer summaries which have been supplied by each title's publisher. Some summaries also include customer reviews. Your local bookseller may have access to in-house and commercial databases that index all published books (e.g. Books in Print®). **IMPORTANT NOTE:** Online booksellers typically produce search results for medical and non-medical books. When searching for "polycystic ovarian syndrome" at online booksellers' Web sites, you may discover non-medical books that use the generic term "polycystic ovarian syndrome" (or a synonym) in their titles. The following is indicative of the results you might find when searching for "polycystic ovarian syndrome" (sorted alphabetically by title; follow the hyperlink to view more details at Amazon.com):

- **Intraovarian Regulators and Polycystic Ovarian Syndrome: Recent Progress on Clinical and Therapeutic Aspects (Annals of the New York Academy of Scie)** by George Tolis, et al; ISBN: 0897667794;
  http://www.amazon.com/exec/obidos/ASIN/0897667794/icongroupinterna

- **Living with P.C.O.S.: Polycystic Ovary Syndrome** by Angela Best-Boss, et al; ISBN: 1886039496;
  http://www.amazon.com/exec/obidos/ASIN/1886039496/icongroupinterna

- **Polycystic Ovarian Disease (Clinical Perspectives in Obstetrics and Gynecology)** by Walter Futterweit; ISBN: 0387909818;
  http://www.amazon.com/exec/obidos/ASIN/0387909818/icongroupinterna

- **What to Do When the Doctor Says It's Pcos: (Polycystic Ovarian Syndrome)** by Cheryl Kimball, et al; ISBN: 1592330045;
  http://www.amazon.com/exec/obidos/ASIN/1592330045/icongroupinterna

The National Library of Medicine Book Index

The National Library of Medicine at the National Institutes of Health has a massive database of books published on healthcare and biomedicine. Go to the following Internet site, **http://locatorplus.gov/**, and then select "Search LOCATORplus." Once you are in the search area, simply type "polycystic ovarian syndrome" (or synonyms) into the search box, and select "books only." From there, results can be sorted by publication date, author, or relevance. The following was recently catalogued by the National Library of Medicine:[11]

- **Gonadotropins, insulin, and androgens in women with polycystic ovarian disease** Author: Anttila, Leena,; Year: 1993; Turku: Turun Yliopisto, 1993; ISBN: 9518809488
- **Polycystic ovarian disease** Author: Katz, Maurice.; Year: 1986; Chicago, IL: Year Book Medical Publishers, c1984
- **Polycystic ovaries: a disorder or a symptom?** Author: Shaw, Robert W. (Robert Wayne); Year: 1991; Carnforth, Lancs, UK; Park Ridge, N.J., USA: Parthenon Pub. Group, 1991; ISBN: 1850703434
  http://www.amazon.com/exec/obidos/ASIN/1850703434/icongroupinterna
- **Polycystic ovary syndrome** Author: Dunaif, Andrea.; Year: 1992; Boston: Blackwell Scientific Publications; St. Louis, Mo.: Distributors, USA and Canada, Mosby-Year Book, 1992; ISBN: 0865421420
  http://www.amazon.com/exec/obidos/ASIN/0865421420/icongroupinterna
- **The polycystic ovary syndrome: some pathophysiological, diagnostical, and therapeutic aspects** Author: Heineman, Maas Jan,; Year: 1984; [Nijmegen?: s.n., 1982?]

Chapters on Polycystic Ovarian Syndrome

In order to find chapters that specifically relate to polycystic ovarian syndrome, an excellent source of abstracts is the Combined Health Information Database. You will need to limit your search to book chapters and polycystic ovarian syndrome using the "Detailed Search" option. Go to the following hyperlink: **http://chid.nih.gov/detail/detail.html**. To find book chapters, use the drop boxes at the bottom of the search page where "You may refine your search by." Select the dates and language you prefer, and the format option "Book Chapter." Type "polycystic ovarian syndrome" (or synonyms) into the "For these words:" box. The following is a typical result when searching for book chapters on polycystic ovarian syndrome:

---

[11] In addition to LOCATORPlus, in collaboration with authors and publishers, the National Center for Biotechnology Information (NCBI) is currently adapting biomedical books for the Web. The books may be accessed in two ways: (1) by searching directly using any search term or phrase (in the same way as the bibliographic database PubMed), or (2) by following the links to PubMed abstracts. Each PubMed abstract has a "Books" button that displays a facsimile of the abstract in which some phrases are hypertext links. These phrases are also found in the books available at NCBI. Click on hyperlinked results in the list of books in which the phrase is found. Currently, the majority of the links are between the books and PubMed. In the future, more links will be created between the books and other types of information, such as gene and protein sequences and macromolecular structures. See **http://www.ncbi.nlm.nih.gov/entrez/query.fcgi?db=Books**.

- **Target Population for Diabetes Prevention: The Metabolically Obese, Normal-Weight Individual**

    Source: in Devlin, J.T. and Schneider, S.H., eds. Handbook of Exercise in Diabetes. Alexandria, VA: American Diabetes Association. 2002. p. 235-249.

    Contact: Available from American Diabetes Association (ADA). Order Fulfillment Department, P.O. Box 930850, Atlanta, GA 31193-0850. (800) 232-6733. Fax (770) 442-9742. Website: www.diabetes.org. PRICE: $69.95 plus shipping and handling. ISBN: 1580400191.

    Summary: Epidemiological evidence suggests that regular physical activity may prevent, or at least retard, the development of type 2 diabetes and coronary heart disease. This benefit of exercise is likely to be most prominent in individuals predisposed to the insulin resistance syndrome. Individuals with insulin resistance often have generalized obesity; however, they also may not be obese or even overweight by present standards. The latter have been referred to as metabolically obese, normal-weight (MONW) individuals. This chapter is from a book that provides a practical, comprehensive guide to diabetes and exercise for health care professionals involved in patient care. In this chapter, the author considers the MONW group as a target population for diabetes prevention. Exercise may be therapeutically more efficacious in MONW individuals than in patients with established type 2 diabetes and overt obesity. People at risk for type 2 diabetes and the insulin resistance syndrome, including MONW individuals, may be identified early by such factors as family history, birth weight, and the presence of gestational diabetes (a type of diabetes that occurs during pregnancy), **polycystic ovarian syndrome,** and central adiposity (the tendency to add fat in the middle of the body). Whether lifestyle modification programs of diet and exercise should be targeted specifically at these high risk individuals or aimed at the general population is a major public health issue. 2 figures. 6 tables. 37 references.

- **New Therapies for Non-Insulin-Dependent Diabetes Mellitus: Thiazolidinediones**

    Source: in LeRoith, D.; Taylor, S.I.; Olefsky, J.M., eds. Diabetes Mellitus: A Fundamental and Clinical Text. Philadelphia, PA: Lippincott-Raven Publishers. 1996. p. 661-668.

    Contact: Available from Lippincott-Raven Publishers. 12107 Insurance Way, Hagerstown, MD 21740-5184. (800) 777-2295. Fax (301) 824-7390. PRICE: $199.00. ISBN: 0397514565.

    Summary: The treatment of noninsulin-dependent diabetes mellitus (NIDDM) has involved the use of insulin or insulin secretagogues such as sulfonylureas or biguanides such as metformin. Although these agents have been effective to a degree, they do not deal directly with the underlying pathology of insulin resistance. This chapter, from a medical textbook on diabetes, describes the use of the thiazolidinediones, a class of drugs that may directly decrease insulin resistance by enhancing insulin action in skeletal muscle, liver, and adipose (fat) tissue. One of these compounds, troglitazone, has progressed to late-stage clinical development. The authors cover how thiazolidinediones improve insulin sensitivity in animal models of diabetes, how these drugs may improve the insulin resistance syndrome, the use of troglitazone in NIDDM, the use of troglitazone in impaired glucose tolerance (IGT), and the potential use of troglitazone in **polycystic ovarian syndrome.** The authors conclude that persons with other insulin-resistant states such as steroid-induced glucose intolerance and severe insulin resistance, as well as women with a history of gestational diabetes, are also populations in whom insulin-sensitizing agents would be valuable, both in treating and potentially preventing hyperglycemic states. 6 figures. 49 references.

Chapter 8. Multimedia on Polycystic Ovarian Syndrome

Overview

In this chapter, we show you how to keep current on multimedia sources of information on polycystic ovarian syndrome. We start with sources that have been summarized by federal agencies, and then show you how to find bibliographic information catalogued by the National Library of Medicine.

Bibliography: Multimedia on Polycystic Ovarian Syndrome

The National Library of Medicine is a rich source of information on healthcare-related multimedia productions including slides, computer software, and databases. To access the multimedia database, go to the following Web site: **http://locatorplus.gov/**. Select "Search LOCATORplus." Once in the search area, simply type in polycystic ovarian syndrome (or synonyms). Then, in the option box provided below the search box, select "Audiovisuals and Computer Files." From there, you can choose to sort results by publication date, author, or relevance. The following multimedia has been indexed on polycystic ovarian syndrome:

- **Polycystic ovary syndrome [slide]** Source: Luther M. Talbert; Year: 1977; Format: Slide; Chapel Hill, N.C.: Health Sciences Consortium, c1977
- **Polycystic ovary syndrome and the androgen-insulin connection [videorecording]** Source: the University of Texas Medical School at Houston; produced by UT-TV, Houston; Year: 1992; Format: Videorecording; [Houston, Tex.: UT-TV], c1992
- **Scrambled [videorecording]: polycystic ovarian syndrome.** Year: 2003; Format: Videorecording; Boston, MA: Fanlight Productions, 2003

Chapter 9. Periodicals and News on Polycystic Ovarian Syndrome

Overview

In this chapter, we suggest a number of news sources and present various periodicals that cover polycystic ovarian syndrome.

News Services and Press Releases

One of the simplest ways of tracking press releases on polycystic ovarian syndrome is to search the news wires. In the following sample of sources, we will briefly describe how to access each service. These services only post recent news intended for public viewing.

PR Newswire

To access the PR Newswire archive, simply go to **http://www.prnewswire.com/**. Select your country. Type "polycystic ovarian syndrome" (or synonyms) into the search box. You will automatically receive information on relevant news releases posted within the last 30 days. The search results are shown by order of relevance.

Reuters Health

The Reuters' Medical News and Health eLine databases can be very useful in exploring news archives relating to polycystic ovarian syndrome. While some of the listed articles are free to view, others are available for purchase for a nominal fee. To access this archive, go to **http://www.reutershealth.com/en/index.html** and search by "polycystic ovarian syndrome" (or synonyms). The following was recently listed in this archive for polycystic ovarian syndrome:

- **Girls with polycystic ovarian syndrome may be at increased risk of type 2 diabetes**
  Source: Reuters Medical News
  Date: February 26, 2001

- **Hyperinsulinemia increases CVD risk in women with polycystic ovarian syndrome**
  Source: Reuters Medical News
  Date: January 10, 2000
- **Recombinant FSH stimulates follicular growth in women with polycystic ovarian syndrome**
  Source: Reuters Medical News
  Date: February 16, 1999

The NIH

Within MEDLINEplus, the NIH has made an agreement with the New York Times Syndicate, the AP News Service, and Reuters to deliver news that can be browsed by the public. Search news releases at **http://www.nlm.nih.gov/medlineplus/alphanews_a.html**. MEDLINEplus allows you to browse across an alphabetical index. Or you can search by date at the following Web page: **http://www.nlm.nih.gov/medlineplus/newsbydate.html**. Often, news items are indexed by MEDLINEplus within its search engine.

Business Wire

Business Wire is similar to PR Newswire. To access this archive, simply go to **http://www.businesswire.com/**. You can scan the news by industry category or company name.

Market Wire

Market Wire is more focused on technology than the other wires. To browse the latest press releases by topic, such as alternative medicine, biotechnology, fitness, healthcare, legal, nutrition, and pharmaceuticals, access Market Wire's Medical/Health channel at **http://www.marketwire.com/mw/release_index?channel=MedicalHealth**. Or simply go to Market Wire's home page at **http://www.marketwire.com/mw/home**, type "polycystic ovarian syndrome" (or synonyms) into the search box, and click on "Search News." As this service is technology oriented, you may wish to use it when searching for press releases covering diagnostic procedures or tests.

Search Engines

Medical news is also available in the news sections of commercial Internet search engines. See the health news page at Yahoo (**http://dir.yahoo.com/Health/News_and_Media/**), or you can use this Web site's general news search page at **http://news.yahoo.com/**. Type in "polycystic ovarian syndrome" (or synonyms). If you know the name of a company that is relevant to polycystic ovarian syndrome, you can go to any stock trading Web site (such as **http://www.etrade.com/**) and search for the company name there. News items across various news sources are reported on indicated hyperlinks. Google offers a similar service at **http://news.google.com/**.

BBC

Covering news from a more European perspective, the British Broadcasting Corporation (BBC) allows the public free access to their news archive located at **http://www.bbc.co.uk/**. Search by "polycystic ovarian syndrome" (or synonyms).

Academic Periodicals covering Polycystic Ovarian Syndrome

Numerous periodicals are currently indexed within the National Library of Medicine's PubMed database that are known to publish articles relating to polycystic ovarian syndrome. In addition to these sources, you can search for articles covering polycystic ovarian syndrome that have been published by any of the periodicals listed in previous chapters. To find the latest studies published, go to **http://www.ncbi.nlm.nih.gov/pubmed**, type the name of the periodical into the search box, and click "Go."

If you want complete details about the historical contents of a journal, you can also visit the following Web site: **http://www.ncbi.nlm.nih.gov/entrez/jrbrowser.cgi**. Here, type in the name of the journal or its abbreviation, and you will receive an index of published articles. At **http://locatorplus.gov/**, you can retrieve more indexing information on medical periodicals (e.g. the name of the publisher). Select the button "Search LOCATORplus." Then type in the name of the journal and select the advanced search option "Journal Title Search."

APPENDICES

APPENDIX A. PHYSICIAN RESOURCES

Overview

In this chapter, we focus on databases and Internet-based guidelines and information resources created or written for a professional audience.

NIH Guidelines

Commonly referred to as "clinical" or "professional" guidelines, the National Institutes of Health publish physician guidelines for the most common diseases. Publications are available at the following by relevant Institute[12]:

- Office of the Director (OD); guidelines consolidated across agencies available at
  http://www.nih.gov/health/consumer/conkey.htm

- National Institute of General Medical Sciences (NIGMS); fact sheets available at
  http://www.nigms.nih.gov/news/facts/

- National Library of Medicine (NLM); extensive encyclopedia (A.D.A.M., Inc.) with guidelines: http://www.nlm.nih.gov/medlineplus/healthtopics.html

- National Cancer Institute (NCI); guidelines available at
  http://www.cancer.gov/cancerinfo/list.aspx?viewid=5f35036e-5497-4d86-8c2c-714a9f7c8d25

- National Eye Institute (NEI); guidelines available at
  http://www.nei.nih.gov/order/index.htm

- National Heart, Lung, and Blood Institute (NHLBI); guidelines available at
  http://www.nhlbi.nih.gov/guidelines/index.htm

- National Human Genome Research Institute (NHGRI); research available at
  http://www.genome.gov/page.cfm?pageID=10000375

- National Institute on Aging (NIA); guidelines available at
  http://www.nia.nih.gov/health/

---

[12] These publications are typically written by one or more of the various NIH Institutes.

- National Institute on Alcohol Abuse and Alcoholism (NIAAA); guidelines available at http://www.niaaa.nih.gov/publications/publications.htm

- National Institute of Allergy and Infectious Diseases (NIAID); guidelines available at http://www.niaid.nih.gov/publications/

- National Institute of Arthritis and Musculoskeletal and Skin Diseases (NIAMS); fact sheets and guidelines available at http://www.niams.nih.gov/hi/index.htm

- National Institute of Child Health and Human Development (NICHD); guidelines available at http://www.nichd.nih.gov/publications/pubskey.cfm

- National Institute on Deafness and Other Communication Disorders (NIDCD); fact sheets and guidelines at http://www.nidcd.nih.gov/health/

- National Institute of Dental and Craniofacial Research (NIDCR); guidelines available at http://www.nidr.nih.gov/health/

- National Institute of Diabetes and Digestive and Kidney Diseases (NIDDK); guidelines available at http://www.niddk.nih.gov/health/health.htm

- National Institute on Drug Abuse (NIDA); guidelines available at http://www.nida.nih.gov/DrugAbuse.html

- National Institute of Environmental Health Sciences (NIEHS); environmental health information available at http://www.niehs.nih.gov/external/facts.htm

- National Institute of Mental Health (NIMH); guidelines available at http://www.nimh.nih.gov/practitioners/index.cfm

- National Institute of Neurological Disorders and Stroke (NINDS); neurological disorder information pages available at http://www.ninds.nih.gov/health_and_medical/disorder_index.htm

- National Institute of Nursing Research (NINR); publications on selected illnesses at http://www.nih.gov/ninr/news-info/publications.html

- National Institute of Biomedical Imaging and Bioengineering; general information at http://grants.nih.gov/grants/becon/becon_info.htm

- Center for Information Technology (CIT); referrals to other agencies based on keyword searches available at http://kb.nih.gov/www_query_main.asp

- National Center for Complementary and Alternative Medicine (NCCAM); health information available at http://nccam.nih.gov/health/

- National Center for Research Resources (NCRR); various information directories available at http://www.ncrr.nih.gov/publications.asp

- Office of Rare Diseases; various fact sheets available at http://rarediseases.info.nih.gov/html/resources/rep_pubs.html

- Centers for Disease Control and Prevention; various fact sheets on infectious diseases available at http://www.cdc.gov/publications.htm

NIH Databases

In addition to the various Institutes of Health that publish professional guidelines, the NIH has designed a number of databases for professionals.[13] Physician-oriented resources provide a wide variety of information related to the biomedical and health sciences, both past and present. The format of these resources varies. Searchable databases, bibliographic citations, full-text articles (when available), archival collections, and images are all available. The following are referenced by the National Library of Medicine:[14]

- **Bioethics:** Access to published literature on the ethical, legal, and public policy issues surrounding healthcare and biomedical research. This information is provided in conjunction with the Kennedy Institute of Ethics located at Georgetown University, Washington, D.C.: http://www.nlm.nih.gov/databases/databases_bioethics.html

- **HIV/AIDS Resources:** Describes various links and databases dedicated to HIV/AIDS research: http://www.nlm.nih.gov/pubs/factsheets/aidsinfs.html

- **NLM Online Exhibitions:** Describes "Exhibitions in the History of Medicine": http://www.nlm.nih.gov/exhibition/exhibition.html. Additional resources for historical scholarship in medicine: http://www.nlm.nih.gov/hmd/hmd.html

- **Biotechnology Information:** Access to public databases. The National Center for Biotechnology Information conducts research in computational biology, develops software tools for analyzing genome data, and disseminates biomedical information for the better understanding of molecular processes affecting human health and disease: http://www.ncbi.nlm.nih.gov/

- **Population Information:** The National Library of Medicine provides access to worldwide coverage of population, family planning, and related health issues, including family planning technology and programs, fertility, and population law and policy: http://www.nlm.nih.gov/databases/databases_population.html

- **Cancer Information:** Access to cancer-oriented databases: http://www.nlm.nih.gov/databases/databases_cancer.html

- **Profiles in Science:** Offering the archival collections of prominent twentieth-century biomedical scientists to the public through modern digital technology: http://www.profiles.nlm.nih.gov/

- **Chemical Information:** Provides links to various chemical databases and references: http://sis.nlm.nih.gov/Chem/ChemMain.html

- **Clinical Alerts:** Reports the release of findings from the NIH-funded clinical trials where such release could significantly affect morbidity and mortality: http://www.nlm.nih.gov/databases/alerts/clinical_alerts.html

- **Space Life Sciences:** Provides links and information to space-based research (including NASA): http://www.nlm.nih.gov/databases/databases_space.html

- **MEDLINE:** Bibliographic database covering the fields of medicine, nursing, dentistry, veterinary medicine, the healthcare system, and the pre-clinical sciences: http://www.nlm.nih.gov/databases/databases_medline.html

---

[13] Remember, for the general public, the National Library of Medicine recommends the databases referenced in MEDLINE*plus* (http://medlineplus.gov/ or http://www.nlm.nih.gov/medlineplus/databases.html).

[14] See http://www.nlm.nih.gov/databases/databases.html.

114 Polycystic Ovarian Syndrome

- **Toxicology and Environmental Health Information (TOXNET):** Databases covering toxicology and environmental health: **http://sis.nlm.nih.gov/Tox/ToxMain.html**
- **Visible Human Interface:** Anatomically detailed, three-dimensional representations of normal male and female human bodies:
  http://www.nlm.nih.gov/research/visible/visible_human.html

The NLM Gateway[15]

The NLM (National Library of Medicine) Gateway is a Web-based system that lets users search simultaneously in multiple retrieval systems at the U.S. National Library of Medicine (NLM). It allows users of NLM services to initiate searches from one Web interface, providing one-stop searching for many of NLM's information resources or databases.[16] To use the NLM Gateway, simply go to the search site at **http://gateway.nlm.nih.gov/gw/Cmd**. Type "polycystic ovarian syndrome" (or synonyms) into the search box and click "Search." The results will be presented in a tabular form, indicating the number of references in each database category.

Results Summary

Category	Items Found
Journal Articles	4680
Books / Periodicals / Audio Visual	36
Consumer Health	468
Meeting Abstracts	3
Other Collections	0
Total	5187

HSTAT[17]

HSTAT is a free, Web-based resource that provides access to full-text documents used in healthcare decision-making.[18] These documents include clinical practice guidelines, quick-reference guides for clinicians, consumer health brochures, evidence reports and technology assessments from the Agency for Healthcare Research and Quality (AHRQ), as well as AHRQ's Put Prevention Into Practice.[19] Simply search by "polycystic ovarian syndrome" (or synonyms) at the following Web site: **http://text.nlm.nih.gov**.

---

[15] Adapted from NLM: **http://gateway.nlm.nih.gov/gw/Cmd?Overview.x**.

[16] The NLM Gateway is currently being developed by the Lister Hill National Center for Biomedical Communications (LHNCBC) at the National Library of Medicine (NLM) of the National Institutes of Health (NIH).

[17] Adapted from HSTAT: **http://www.nlm.nih.gov/pubs/factsheets/hstat.html**.

[18] The HSTAT URL is **http://hstat.nlm.nih.gov/**.

[19] Other important documents in HSTAT include: the National Institutes of Health (NIH) Consensus Conference Reports and Technology Assessment Reports; the HIV/AIDS Treatment Information Service (ATIS) resource documents; the Substance Abuse and Mental Health Services Administration's Center for Substance Abuse Treatment (SAMHSA/CSAT) Treatment Improvement Protocols (TIP) and Center for Substance Abuse Prevention (SAMHSA/CSAP) Prevention Enhancement Protocols System (PEPS); the Public Health Service (PHS) Preventive Services Task Force's *Guide to Clinical Preventive Services*; the independent, nonfederal Task Force on Community Services' *Guide to Community Preventive Services*; and the Health Technology Advisory Committee (HTAC) of the Minnesota Health Care Commission (MHCC) health technology evaluations.

Coffee Break: Tutorials for Biologists [20]

Coffee Break is a general healthcare site that takes a scientific view of the news and covers recent breakthroughs in biology that may one day assist physicians in developing treatments. Here you will find a collection of short reports on recent biological discoveries. Each report incorporates interactive tutorials that demonstrate how bioinformatics tools are used as a part of the research process. Currently, all Coffee Breaks are written by NCBI staff.[21] Each report is about 400 words and is usually based on a discovery reported in one or more articles from recently published, peer-reviewed literature.[22] This site has new articles every few weeks, so it can be considered an online magazine of sorts. It is intended for general background information. You can access the Coffee Break Web site at the following hyperlink: **http://www.ncbi.nlm.nih.gov/Coffeebreak/**.

Other Commercial Databases

In addition to resources maintained by official agencies, other databases exist that are commercial ventures addressing medical professionals. Here are some examples that may interest you:

- **CliniWeb International:** Index and table of contents to selected clinical information on the Internet; see **http://www.ohsu.edu/cliniweb/**.

- **Medical World Search:** Searches full text from thousands of selected medical sites on the Internet; see **http://www.mwsearch.com/**.

The Genome Project and Polycystic Ovarian Syndrome

In the following section, we will discuss databases and references which relate to the Genome Project and polycystic ovarian syndrome.

Online Mendelian Inheritance in Man (OMIM)

The Online Mendelian Inheritance in Man (OMIM) database is a catalog of human genes and genetic disorders authored and edited by Dr. Victor A. McKusick and his colleagues at Johns Hopkins and elsewhere. OMIM was developed for the World Wide Web by the National Center for Biotechnology Information (NCBI).[23] The database contains textual information, pictures, and reference information. It also contains copious links to NCBI's Entrez database of MEDLINE articles and sequence information.

---

[20] Adapted from http://www.ncbi.nlm.nih.gov/Coffeebreak/Archive/FAQ.html.

[21] The figure that accompanies each article is frequently supplied by an expert external to NCBI, in which case the source of the figure is cited. The result is an interactive tutorial that tells a biological story.

[22] After a brief introduction that sets the work described into a broader context, the report focuses on how a molecular understanding can provide explanations of observed biology and lead to therapies for diseases. Each vignette is accompanied by a figure and hypertext links that lead to a series of pages that interactively show how NCBI tools and resources are used in the research process.

[23] Adapted from http://www.ncbi.nlm.nih.gov/. Established in 1988 as a national resource for molecular biology information, NCBI creates public databases, conducts research in computational biology, develops software tools for analyzing genome data, and disseminates biomedical information--all for the better understanding of molecular processes affecting human health and disease.

To search the database, go to **http://www.ncbi.nlm.nih.gov/Omim/searchomim.html**. Type "polycystic ovarian syndrome" (or synonyms) into the search box, and click "Submit Search." If too many results appear, you can narrow the search by adding the word "clinical." Each report will have additional links to related research and databases. In particular, the option "Database Links" will search across technical databases that offer an abundance of information. The following is an example of the results you can obtain from the OMIM for polycystic ovarian syndrome:

- **Polycystic Ovary Syndrome 1**
  Web site: http://www.ncbi.nlm.nih.gov/htbin-post/Omim/dispmim?184700

Genes and Disease (NCBI - Map)

The Genes and Disease database is produced by the National Center for Biotechnology Information of the National Library of Medicine at the National Institutes of Health. This Web site categorizes each disorder by system of the body. Go to **http://www.ncbi.nlm.nih.gov/disease/**, and browse the system pages to have a full view of important conditions linked to human genes. Since this site is regularly updated, you may wish to revisit it from time to time. The following systems and associated disorders are addressed:

- **Cancer:** Uncontrolled cell division.
  Examples: Breast and ovarian cancer, Burkitt lymphoma, chronic myeloid leukemia, colon cancer, lung cancer, malignant melanoma, multiple endocrine neoplasia, neurofibromatosis, p53 tumor suppressor, pancreatic cancer, prostate cancer, Ras oncogene, RB: retinoblastoma, von Hippel-Lindau syndrome.
  Web site: **http://www.ncbi.nlm.nih.gov/disease/Cancer.html**

- **Immune System:** Fights invaders.
  Examples: Asthma, autoimmune polyglandular syndrome, Crohn's disease, DiGeorge syndrome, familial Mediterranean fever, immunodeficiency with Hyper-IgM, severe combined immunodeficiency.
  Web site: **http://www.ncbi.nlm.nih.gov/disease/Immune.html**

- **Metabolism:** Food and energy.
  Examples: Adreno-leukodystrophy, atherosclerosis, Best disease, Gaucher disease, glucose galactose malabsorption, gyrate atrophy, juvenile-onset diabetes, obesity, paroxysmal nocturnal hemoglobinuria, phenylketonuria, Refsum disease, Tangier disease, Tay-Sachs disease.
  Web site: **http://www.ncbi.nlm.nih.gov/disease/Metabolism.html**

- **Muscle and Bone:** Movement and growth.
  Examples: Duchenne muscular dystrophy, Ellis-van Creveld syndrome, Marfan syndrome, myotonic dystrophy, spinal muscular atrophy.
  Web site: **http://www.ncbi.nlm.nih.gov/disease/Muscle.html**

- **Nervous System:** Mind and body.
  Examples: Alzheimer disease, amyotrophic lateral sclerosis, Angelman syndrome, Charcot-Marie-Tooth disease, epilepsy, essential tremor, fragile X syndrome, Friedreich's ataxia, Huntington disease, Niemann-Pick disease, Parkinson disease, Prader-Willi syndrome, Rett syndrome, spinocerebellar atrophy, Williams syndrome.
  Web site: **http://www.ncbi.nlm.nih.gov/disease/Brain.html**

- **Signals:** Cellular messages.
  Examples: Ataxia telangiectasia, Cockayne syndrome, glaucoma, male-patterned baldness, SRY: sex determination, tuberous sclerosis, Waardenburg syndrome, Werner syndrome.
  Web site: http://www.ncbi.nlm.nih.gov/disease/Signals.html
- **Transporters:** Pumps and channels.
  Examples: Cystic fibrosis, deafness, diastrophic dysplasia, Hemophilia A, long-QT syndrome, Menkes syndrome, Pendred syndrome, polycystic kidney disease, sickle cell anemia, Wilson's disease, Zellweger syndrome.
  Web site: http://www.ncbi.nlm.nih.gov/disease/Transporters.html

Entrez

Entrez is a search and retrieval system that integrates several linked databases at the National Center for Biotechnology Information (NCBI). These databases include nucleotide sequences, protein sequences, macromolecular structures, whole genomes, and MEDLINE through PubMed. Entrez provides access to the following databases:

- **3D Domains:** Domains from Entrez Structure,
  Web site: http://www.ncbi.nlm.nih.gov/entrez/query.fcgi?db=geo
- **Books:** Online books,
  Web site: http://www.ncbi.nlm.nih.gov/entrez/query.fcgi?db=books
- **Genome:** Complete genome assemblies,
  Web site: http://www.ncbi.nlm.nih.gov/entrez/query.fcgi?db=Genome
- **NCBI's Protein Sequence Information Survey Results:**
  Web site: http://www.ncbi.nlm.nih.gov/About/proteinsurvey/
- **Nucleotide Sequence Database (Genbank):**
  Web site: http://www.ncbi.nlm.nih.gov/entrez/query.fcgi?db=Nucleotide
- **OMIM:** Online Mendelian Inheritance in Man,
  Web site: http://www.ncbi.nlm.nih.gov/entrez/query.fcgi?db=OMIM
- **PopSet:** Population study data sets,
  Web site: http://www.ncbi.nlm.nih.gov/entrez/query.fcgi?db=Popset
- **ProbeSet:** Gene Expression Omnibus (GEO),
  Web site: http://www.ncbi.nlm.nih.gov/entrez/query.fcgi?db=geo
- **Protein Sequence Database:**
  Web site: http://www.ncbi.nlm.nih.gov/entrez/query.fcgi?db=Protein
- **PubMed:** Biomedical literature (PubMed),
  Web site: http://www.ncbi.nlm.nih.gov/entrez/query.fcgi?db=PubMed
- **Structure:** Three-dimensional macromolecular structures,
  Web site: http://www.ncbi.nlm.nih.gov/entrez/query.fcgi?db=Structure
- **Taxonomy:** Organisms in GenBank,
  Web site: http://www.ncbi.nlm.nih.gov/entrez/query.fcgi?db=Taxonomy

To access the Entrez system at the National Center for Biotechnology Information, go to http://www.ncbi.nlm.nih.gov/entrez/query.fcgi?CMD=search&DB=genome, and then select the database that you would like to search. The databases available are listed in the drop box next to "Search." Enter "polycystic ovarian syndrome" (or synonyms) into the search box and click "Go."

Jablonski's Multiple Congenital Anomaly/Mental Retardation (MCA/MR) Syndromes Database[24]

This online resource has been developed to facilitate the identification and differentiation of syndromic entities. Special attention is given to the type of information that is usually limited or completely omitted in existing reference sources due to space limitations of the printed form.

At **http://www.nlm.nih.gov/mesh/jablonski/syndrome_toc/toc_a.html**, you can search across syndromes using an alphabetical index. Search by keywords at **http://www.nlm.nih.gov/mesh/jablonski/syndrome_db.html**.

The Genome Database[25]

Established at Johns Hopkins University in Baltimore, Maryland in 1990, the Genome Database (GDB) is the official central repository for genomic mapping data resulting from the Human Genome Initiative. In the spring of 1999, the Bioinformatics Supercomputing Centre (BiSC) at the Hospital for Sick Children in Toronto, Ontario assumed the management of GDB. The Human Genome Initiative is a worldwide research effort focusing on structural analysis of human DNA to determine the location and sequence of the estimated 100,000 human genes. In support of this project, GDB stores and curates data generated by researchers worldwide who are engaged in the mapping effort of the Human Genome Project (HGP). GDB's mission is to provide scientists with an encyclopedia of the human genome which is continually revised and updated to reflect the current state of scientific knowledge. Although GDB has historically focused on gene mapping, its focus will broaden as the Genome Project moves from mapping to sequence, and finally, to functional analysis.

To access the GDB, simply go to the following hyperlink: **http://www.gdb.org/**. Search "All Biological Data" by "Keyword." Type "polycystic ovarian syndrome" (or synonyms) into the search box, and review the results. If more than one word is used in the search box, then separate each one with the word "and" or "or" (using "or" might be useful when using synonyms).

---

[24] Adapted from the National Library of Medicine: http://www.nlm.nih.gov/mesh/jablonski/about_syndrome.html.

[25] Adapted from the Genome Database: http://gdbwww.gdb.org/gdb/aboutGDB.html - mission.

APPENDIX B. PATIENT RESOURCES

Overview

Official agencies, as well as federally funded institutions supported by national grants, frequently publish a variety of guidelines written with the patient in mind. These are typically called "Fact Sheets" or "Guidelines." They can take the form of a brochure, information kit, pamphlet, or flyer. Often they are only a few pages in length. Since new guidelines on polycystic ovarian syndrome can appear at any moment and be published by a number of sources, the best approach to finding guidelines is to systematically scan the Internet-based services that post them.

Patient Guideline Sources

The remainder of this chapter directs you to sources which either publish or can help you find additional guidelines on topics related to polycystic ovarian syndrome. Due to space limitations, these sources are listed in a concise manner. Do not hesitate to consult the following sources by either using the Internet hyperlink provided, or, in cases where the contact information is provided, contacting the publisher or author directly.

The National Institutes of Health

The NIH gateway to patients is located at **http://health.nih.gov/**. From this site, you can search across various sources and institutes, a number of which are summarized below.

Topic Pages: MEDLINEplus

The National Library of Medicine has created a vast and patient-oriented healthcare information portal called MEDLINEplus. Within this Internet-based system are "health topic pages" which list links to available materials relevant to polycystic ovarian syndrome. To access this system, log on to **http://www.nlm.nih.gov/medlineplus/healthtopics.html**. From there you can either search using the alphabetical index or browse by broad topic areas. Recently, MEDLINEplus listed the following when searched for "polycystic ovarian syndrome":

120 Polycystic Ovarian Syndrome

- Other guides

    Hormones
    http://www.nlm.nih.gov/medlineplus/hormones.html

    Infertility
    http://www.nlm.nih.gov/medlineplus/infertility.html

    Kidney Diseases
    http://www.nlm.nih.gov/medlineplus/kidneydiseases.html

    Menstruation and Premenstrual Syndrome
    http://www.nlm.nih.gov/medlineplus/menstruationandpremenstrualsyndrome.html

    Ovarian Cancer
    http://www.nlm.nih.gov/medlineplus/ovariancancer.html

    Ovarian Cancer
    http://www.nlm.nih.gov/medlineplus/tutorials/whatisovariancancerloader.html

    Ovarian Cysts
    http://www.nlm.nih.gov/medlineplus/ovariancysts.html

    Reproductive Health
    http://www.nlm.nih.gov/medlineplus/reproductivehealth.html

    Uterine Cancer
    http://www.nlm.nih.gov/medlineplus/uterinecancer.html

    Uterine Diseases
    http://www.nlm.nih.gov/medlineplus/uterinediseases.html

    Vaginal Diseases
    http://www.nlm.nih.gov/medlineplus/vaginaldiseases.html

Within the health topic page dedicated to polycystic ovarian syndrome, the following was listed:

- General/Overviews

    Ovarian Cysts
    http://www.nlm.nih.gov/medlineplus/tutorials/ovariancystsloader.html

    Ovarian Cysts
    Source: American College of Obstetricians and Gynecologists
    http://www.medem.com/medlb/article_detaillb.cfm?article_ID=ZZZEB8EN97C&sub_cat=9

    Ovarian Cysts
    Source: Mayo Foundation for Medical Education and Research
    http://www.mayoclinic.com/invoke.cfm?id=DS00129

- Diagnosis/Symptoms

    Laparoscopy
    Source: American College of Obstetricians and Gynecologists
    http://www.medem.com/MedLB/article_detaillb.cfm?article_ID=ZZZODAA697C

&sub_cat=8

Polycystic Ovary Syndrome Frequently Asked Questions: Diagnosing PCOS
Source: International Council on Infertility Information Dissemination
http://www.inciid.org/faq/pcos2.html

Ultrasound-Pelvis
Source: American College of Radiology, Radiological Society of North America
http://www.radiologyinfo.org/content/ultrasound-pelvis.htm

- Treatment

    Polycystic Ovary Syndrome Frequently Asked Questions: Treating Infertility Due to PCOS
    Source: International Council on Infertility Information Dissemination
    http://www.inciid.org/faq/pcos5.html

    Polycystic Ovary Syndrome Frequently Asked Questions: Treating PCOS When Not Trying to Conceive
    Source: International Council on Infertility Information Dissemination
    http://www.inciid.org/faq/pcos8.html

- Specific Conditions/Aspects

    Hemorrhagic Cysts in the Ovary
    Source: Mayo Foundation for Medical Education and Research
    http://www.mayoclinic.com/invoke.cfm?id=AN00485

    Insulin Resistance Syndrome
    Source: American Academy of Family Physicians
    http://familydoctor.org/660.xml

    Polycystic Ovary Syndrome
    Source: Mayo Foundation for Medical Education and Research
    http://www.mayoclinic.com/invoke.cfm?id=DS00423

    Polycystic Ovary Syndrome Frequently Asked Questions: Cosmetic Concerns
    Source: International Council on Infertility Information Dissemination
    http://www.inciid.org/faq/pcos10.html

    Polycystic Ovary Syndrome Frequently Asked Questions: Emotionally Speaking
    Source: Polycystic Ovarian Syndrome Association
    http://www.inciid.org/faq/pcos11.html

    Polycystic Ovary Syndrome Frequently Asked Questions: Increased Miscarriage Rate with PCOS
    Source: Polycystic Ovarian Syndrome Association
    http://www.inciid.org/faq/pcos6.html

    Polycystic Ovary Syndrome Frequently Asked Questions: Pregnancy with PCOS
    Source: Polycystic Ovarian Syndrome Association
    http://www.inciid.org/faq/pcos7.html

    Polycystic Ovary Syndrome Frequently Asked Questions: The Insulin Connection and How to Treat It
    Source: International Council on Infertility Information Dissemination
    http://www.inciid.org/faq/pcos4.html

Polycystic Ovary Syndrome Frequently Asked Questions: The Syndrome and the Symptoms
Source: International Council on Infertility Information Dissemination
http://www.inciid.org/faq/pcos1.html

Polycystic Ovary Syndrome Frequently Asked Questions: Weight, Diet & Exercise for Women with PCOS
Source: International Council on Infertility Information Dissemination
http://www.inciid.org/faq/pcos9.html

- Organizations

    International Council on Infertility Information Dissemination
    http://www.inciid.org/

    National Institute of Child Health and Human Development
    http://www.nichd.nih.gov/

    National Women's Health Information Center
    Source: Dept. of Health and Human Services
    http://www.4woman.gov/

- Pictures/Diagrams

    Atlas of the Body: Female Reproductive Organs
    Source: American Medical Association
    http://www.medem.com/MedLb/article_detaillb.cfm?article_ID=ZZZ8QKJ56JC&sub_cat=2

- Research

    Oral Diabetes Drug Shows Promise in Preventing Miscarriage in Common Infertility
    Source: National Institute of Child Health and Human Development
    http://www.nih.gov/news/pr/feb2002/nichd-27.htm

- Teenagers

    Coping with Polycystic Ovary Syndrome
    Source: Nemours Foundation
    http://kidshealth.org/teen/sexual_health/girls/pcos.html

You may also choose to use the search utility provided by MEDLINEplus at the following Web address: **http://www.nlm.nih.gov/medlineplus/**. Simply type a keyword into the search box and click "Search." This utility is similar to the NIH search utility, with the exception that it only includes materials that are linked within the MEDLINEplus system (mostly patient-oriented information). It also has the disadvantage of generating unstructured results. We recommend, therefore, that you use this method only if you have a very targeted search.

Healthfinder™

Healthfinder™ is sponsored by the U.S. Department of Health and Human Services and offers links to hundreds of other sites that contain healthcare information. This Web site is located at **http://www.healthfinder.gov**. Again, keyword searches can be used to find guidelines. The following was recently found in this database:

- **Polycystic Ovarian Syndrome Quiz**

    Summary: Women can take this quiz to see if symptoms they have could indicate polycystic ovarian syndrome. This quiz is intended for educational and informational purposes only.

    Source: Polycystic Ovarian Syndrome Association

    http://www.healthfinder.gov/scripts/recordpass.asp?RecordType=0&RecordID=6002

The NIH Search Utility

The NIH search utility allows you to search for documents on over 100 selected Web sites that comprise the NIH-WEB-SPACE. Each of these servers is "crawled" and indexed on an ongoing basis. Your search will produce a list of various documents, all of which will relate in some way to polycystic ovarian syndrome. The drawbacks of this approach are that the information is not organized by theme and that the references are often a mix of information for professionals and patients. Nevertheless, a large number of the listed Web sites provide useful background information. We can only recommend this route, therefore, for relatively rare or specific disorders, or when using highly targeted searches. To use the NIH search utility, visit the following Web page: **http://search.nih.gov/index.html**

Additional Web Sources

A number of Web sites are available to the public that often link to government sites. These can also point you in the direction of essential information. The following is a representative sample:

- AOL: **http://search.aol.com/cat.adp?id=168&layer=&from=subcats**
- Family Village: **http://www.familyvillage.wisc.edu/specific.htm**
- Google: **http://directory.google.com/Top/Health/Conditions_and_Diseases/**
- Med Help International: **http://www.medhelp.org/HealthTopics/A.html**
- Open Directory Project: **http://dmoz.org/Health/Conditions_and_Diseases/**
- Yahoo.com: **http://dir.yahoo.com/Health/Diseases_and_Conditions/**
- WebMD®Health: **http://my.webmd.com/health_topics**

Finding Associations

There are several Internet directories that provide lists of medical associations with information on or resources relating to polycystic ovarian syndrome. By consulting all of associations listed in this chapter, you will have nearly exhausted all sources for patient associations concerned with polycystic ovarian syndrome.

The National Health Information Center (NHIC)

The National Health Information Center (NHIC) offers a free referral service to help people find organizations that provide information about polycystic ovarian syndrome. For more information, see the NHIC's Web site at **http://www.health.gov/NHIC/** or contact an information specialist by calling 1-800-336-4797.

Directory of Health Organizations

The Directory of Health Organizations, provided by the National Library of Medicine Specialized Information Services, is a comprehensive source of information on associations. The Directory of Health Organizations database can be accessed via the Internet at **http://www.sis.nlm.nih.gov/Dir/DirMain.html**. It is composed of two parts: DIRLINE and Health Hotlines.

The DIRLINE database comprises some 10,000 records of organizations, research centers, and government institutes and associations that primarily focus on health and biomedicine. To access DIRLINE directly, go to the following Web site: **http://dirline.nlm.nih.gov/**. Simply type in "polycystic ovarian syndrome" (or a synonym), and you will receive information on all relevant organizations listed in the database.

Health Hotlines directs you to toll-free numbers to over 300 organizations. You can access this database directly at **http://www.sis.nlm.nih.gov/hotlines/**. On this page, you are given the option to search by keyword or by browsing the subject list. When you have received your search results, click on the name of the organization for its description and contact information.

The Combined Health Information Database

Another comprehensive source of information on healthcare associations is the Combined Health Information Database. Using the "Detailed Search" option, you will need to limit your search to "Organizations" and "polycystic ovarian syndrome". Type the following hyperlink into your Web browser: **http://chid.nih.gov/detail/detail.html**. To find associations, use the drop boxes at the bottom of the search page where "You may refine your search by." For publication date, select "All Years." Then, select your preferred language and the format option "Organization Resource Sheet." Type "polycystic ovarian syndrome" (or synonyms) into the "For these words:" box. You should check back periodically with this database since it is updated every three months.

The National Organization for Rare Disorders, Inc.

The National Organization for Rare Disorders, Inc. has prepared a Web site that provides, at no charge, lists of associations organized by health topic. You can access this database at the following Web site: **http://www.rarediseases.org/search/orgsearch.html**. Type "polycystic ovarian syndrome" (or a synonym) into the search box, and click "Submit Query."

APPENDIX C. FINDING MEDICAL LIBRARIES

Overview

In this Appendix, we show you how to quickly find a medical library in your area.

Preparation

Your local public library and medical libraries have interlibrary loan programs with the National Library of Medicine (NLM), one of the largest medical collections in the world. According to the NLM, most of the literature in the general and historical collections of the National Library of Medicine is available on interlibrary loan to any library. If you would like to access NLM medical literature, then visit a library in your area that can request the publications for you.[26]

Finding a Local Medical Library

The quickest method to locate medical libraries is to use the Internet-based directory published by the National Network of Libraries of Medicine (NN/LM). This network includes 4626 members and affiliates that provide many services to librarians, health professionals, and the public. To find a library in your area, simply visit **http://nnlm.gov/members/adv.html** or call 1-800-338-7657.

Medical Libraries in the U.S. and Canada

In addition to the NN/LM, the National Library of Medicine (NLM) lists a number of libraries with reference facilities that are open to the public. The following is the NLM's list and includes hyperlinks to each library's Web site. These Web pages can provide information on hours of operation and other restrictions. The list below is a small sample of

---

[26] Adapted from the NLM: **http://www.nlm.nih.gov/psd/cas/interlibrary.html**.

libraries recommended by the National Library of Medicine (sorted alphabetically by name of the U.S. state or Canadian province where the library is located)[27]:

- **Alabama:** Health InfoNet of Jefferson County (Jefferson County Library Cooperative, Lister Hill Library of the Health Sciences), **http://www.uab.edu/infonet/**
- **Alabama:** Richard M. Scrushy Library (American Sports Medicine Institute)
- **Arizona:** Samaritan Regional Medical Center: The Learning Center (Samaritan Health System, Phoenix, Arizona), **http://www.samaritan.edu/library/bannerlibs.htm**
- **California:** Kris Kelly Health Information Center (St. Joseph Health System, Humboldt), **http://www.humboldt1.com/~kkhic/index.html**
- **California:** Community Health Library of Los Gatos, **http://www.healthlib.org/orgresources.html**
- **California:** Consumer Health Program and Services (CHIPS)(County of Los Angeles Public Library, Los Angeles County Harbor-UCLA Medical Center Library) - Carson, CA, **http://www.colapublib.org/services/chips.html**
- **California:** Gateway Health Library (Sutter Gould Medical Foundation)
- **California:** Health Library (Stanford University Medical Center), **http://www-med.stanford.edu/healthlibrary/**
- **California:** Patient Education Resource Center - Health Information and Resources (University of California, San Francisco), **http://sfghdean.ucsf.edu/barnett/PERC/default.asp**
- **California:** Redwood Health Library (Petaluma Health Care District), **http://www.phcd.org/rdwdlib.html**
- **California:** Los Gatos PlaneTree Health Library, **http://planetreesanjose.org/**
- **California:** Sutter Resource Library (Sutter Hospitals Foundation, Sacramento), **http://suttermedicalcenter.org/library/**
- **California:** Health Sciences Libraries (University of California, Davis), **http://www.lib.ucdavis.edu/healthsci/**
- **California:** ValleyCare Health Library & Ryan Comer Cancer Resource Center (ValleyCare Health System, Pleasanton), **http://gaelnet.stmarys-ca.edu/other.libs/gbal/east/vchl.html**
- **California:** Washington Community Health Resource Library (Fremont), **http://www.healthlibrary.org/**
- **Colorado:** William V. Gervasini Memorial Library (Exempla Healthcare), **http://www.saintjosephdenver.org/yourhealth/libraries/**
- **Connecticut:** Hartford Hospital Health Science Libraries (Hartford Hospital), **http://www.harthosp.org/library/**
- **Connecticut:** Healthnet: Connecticut Consumer Health Information Center (University of Connecticut Health Center, Lyman Maynard Stowe Library), **http://library.uchc.edu/departm/hnet/**

---

[27] Abstracted from **http://www.nlm.nih.gov/medlineplus/libraries.html**.

- **Connecticut:** Waterbury Hospital Health Center Library (Waterbury Hospital, Waterbury), **http://www.waterburyhospital.com/library/consumer.shtml**
- **Delaware:** Consumer Health Library (Christiana Care Health System, Eugene du Pont Preventive Medicine & Rehabilitation Institute, Wilmington), **http://www.christianacare.org/health_guide/health_guide_pmri_health_info.cfm**
- **Delaware:** Lewis B. Flinn Library (Delaware Academy of Medicine, Wilmington), **http://www.delamed.org/chls.html**
- **Georgia:** Family Resource Library (Medical College of Georgia, Augusta), **http://cmc.mcg.edu/kids_families/fam_resources/fam_res_lib/frl.htm**
- **Georgia:** Health Resource Center (Medical Center of Central Georgia, Macon), **http://www.mccg.org/hrc/hrchome.asp**
- **Hawaii:** Hawaii Medical Library: Consumer Health Information Service (Hawaii Medical Library, Honolulu), **http://hml.org/CHIS/**
- **Idaho:** DeArmond Consumer Health Library (Kootenai Medical Center, Coeur d'Alene), **http://www.nicon.org/DeArmond/index.htm**
- **Illinois:** Health Learning Center of Northwestern Memorial Hospital (Chicago), **http://www.nmh.org/health_info/hlc.html**
- **Illinois:** Medical Library (OSF Saint Francis Medical Center, Peoria), **http://www.osfsaintfrancis.org/general/library/**
- **Kentucky:** Medical Library - Services for Patients, Families, Students & the Public (Central Baptist Hospital, Lexington), **http://www.centralbap.com/education/community/library.cfm**
- **Kentucky:** University of Kentucky - Health Information Library (Chandler Medical Center, Lexington), **http://www.mc.uky.edu/PatientEd/**
- **Louisiana:** Alton Ochsner Medical Foundation Library (Alton Ochsner Medical Foundation, New Orleans), **http://www.ochsner.org/library/**
- **Louisiana:** Louisiana State University Health Sciences Center Medical Library-Shreveport, **http://lib-sh.lsuhsc.edu/**
- **Maine:** Franklin Memorial Hospital Medical Library (Franklin Memorial Hospital, Farmington), **http://www.fchn.org/fmh/lib.htm**
- **Maine:** Gerrish-True Health Sciences Library (Central Maine Medical Center, Lewiston), **http://www.cmmc.org/library/library.html**
- **Maine:** Hadley Parrot Health Science Library (Eastern Maine Healthcare, Bangor), **http://www.emh.org/hll/hpl/guide.htm**
- **Maine:** Maine Medical Center Library (Maine Medical Center, Portland), **http://www.mmc.org/library/**
- **Maine:** Parkview Hospital (Brunswick), **http://www.parkviewhospital.org/**
- **Maine:** Southern Maine Medical Center Health Sciences Library (Southern Maine Medical Center, Biddeford), **http://www.smmc.org/services/service.php3?choice=10**
- **Maine:** Stephens Memorial Hospital's Health Information Library (Western Maine Health, Norway), **http://www.wmhcc.org/Library/**

- **Manitoba, Canada:** Consumer & Patient Health Information Service (University of Manitoba Libraries),
  http://www.umanitoba.ca/libraries/units/health/reference/chis.html
- **Manitoba, Canada:** J.W. Crane Memorial Library (Deer Lodge Centre, Winnipeg),
  http://www.deerlodge.mb.ca/crane_library/about.asp
- **Maryland:** Health Information Center at the Wheaton Regional Library (Montgomery County, Dept. of Public Libraries, Wheaton Regional Library),
  http://www.mont.lib.md.us/healthinfo/hic.asp
- **Massachusetts:** Baystate Medical Center Library (Baystate Health System),
  http://www.baystatehealth.com/1024/
- **Massachusetts:** Boston University Medical Center Alumni Medical Library (Boston University Medical Center), http://med-libwww.bu.edu/library/lib.html
- **Massachusetts:** Lowell General Hospital Health Sciences Library (Lowell General Hospital, Lowell), http://www.lowellgeneral.org/library/HomePageLinks/WWW.htm
- **Massachusetts:** Paul E. Woodard Health Sciences Library (New England Baptist Hospital, Boston), http://www.nebh.org/health_lib.asp
- **Massachusetts:** St. Luke's Hospital Health Sciences Library (St. Luke's Hospital, Southcoast Health System, New Bedford), http://www.southcoast.org/library/
- **Massachusetts:** Treadwell Library Consumer Health Reference Center (Massachusetts General Hospital), http://www.mgh.harvard.edu/library/chrcindex.html
- **Massachusetts:** UMass HealthNet (University of Massachusetts Medical School, Worchester), http://healthnet.umassmed.edu/
- **Michigan:** Botsford General Hospital Library - Consumer Health (Botsford General Hospital, Library & Internet Services), http://www.botsfordlibrary.org/consumer.htm
- **Michigan:** Helen DeRoy Medical Library (Providence Hospital and Medical Centers), http://www.providence-hospital.org/library/
- **Michigan:** Marquette General Hospital - Consumer Health Library (Marquette General Hospital, Health Information Center), http://www.mgh.org/center.html
- **Michigan:** Patient Education Resouce Center - University of Michigan Cancer Center (University of Michigan Comprehensive Cancer Center, Ann Arbor),
  http://www.cancer.med.umich.edu/learn/leares.htm
- **Michigan:** Sladen Library & Center for Health Information Resources - Consumer Health Information (Detroit), http://www.henryford.com/body.cfm?id=39330
- **Montana:** Center for Health Information (St. Patrick Hospital and Health Sciences Center, Missoula)
- **National:** Consumer Health Library Directory (Medical Library Association, Consumer and Patient Health Information Section), http://caphis.mlanet.org/directory/index.html
- **National:** National Network of Libraries of Medicine (National Library of Medicine) - provides library services for health professionals in the United States who do not have access to a medical library, http://nnlm.gov/
- **National:** NN/LM List of Libraries Serving the Public (National Network of Libraries of Medicine), http://nnlm.gov/members/

- **Nevada:** Health Science Library, West Charleston Library (Las Vegas-Clark County Library District, Las Vegas), http://www.lvccld.org/special_collections/medical/index.htm
- **New Hampshire:** Dartmouth Biomedical Libraries (Dartmouth College Library, Hanover), http://www.dartmouth.edu/~biomed/resources.htmld/conshealth.htmld/
- **New Jersey:** Consumer Health Library (Rahway Hospital, Rahway), http://www.rahwayhospital.com/library.htm
- **New Jersey:** Dr. Walter Phillips Health Sciences Library (Englewood Hospital and Medical Center, Englewood), http://www.englewoodhospital.com/links/index.htm
- **New Jersey:** Meland Foundation (Englewood Hospital and Medical Center, Englewood), http://www.geocities.com/ResearchTriangle/9360/
- **New York:** Choices in Health Information (New York Public Library) - NLM Consumer Pilot Project participant, http://www.nypl.org/branch/health/links.html
- **New York:** Health Information Center (Upstate Medical University, State University of New York, Syracuse), http://www.upstate.edu/library/hic/
- **New York:** Health Sciences Library (Long Island Jewish Medical Center, New Hyde Park), http://www.lij.edu/library/library.html
- **New York:** ViaHealth Medical Library (Rochester General Hospital), http://www.nyam.org/library/
- **Ohio:** Consumer Health Library (Akron General Medical Center, Medical & Consumer Health Library), http://www.akrongeneral.org/hwlibrary.htm
- **Oklahoma:** The Health Information Center at Saint Francis Hospital (Saint Francis Health System, Tulsa), http://www.sfh-tulsa.com/services/healthinfo.asp
- **Oregon:** Planetree Health Resource Center (Mid-Columbia Medical Center, The Dalles), http://www.mcmc.net/phrc/
- **Pennsylvania:** Community Health Information Library (Milton S. Hershey Medical Center, Hershey), http://www.hmc.psu.edu/commhealth/
- **Pennsylvania:** Community Health Resource Library (Geisinger Medical Center, Danville), http://www.geisinger.edu/education/commlib.shtml
- **Pennsylvania:** HealthInfo Library (Moses Taylor Hospital, Scranton), http://www.mth.org/healthwellness.html
- **Pennsylvania:** Hopwood Library (University of Pittsburgh, Health Sciences Library System, Pittsburgh), http://www.hsls.pitt.edu/guides/chi/hopwood/index_html
- **Pennsylvania:** Koop Community Health Information Center (College of Physicians of Philadelphia), http://www.collphyphil.org/kooppg1.shtml
- **Pennsylvania:** Learning Resources Center - Medical Library (Susquehanna Health System, Williamsport), http://www.shscares.org/services/lrc/index.asp
- **Pennsylvania:** Medical Library (UPMC Health System, Pittsburgh), http://www.upmc.edu/passavant/library.htm
- **Quebec, Canada:** Medical Library (Montreal General Hospital), http://www.mghlib.mcgill.ca/

- **South Dakota:** Rapid City Regional Hospital Medical Library (Rapid City Regional Hospital), **http://www.rcrh.org/Services/Library/Default.asp**
- **Texas:** Houston HealthWays (Houston Academy of Medicine-Texas Medical Center Library), **http://hhw.library.tmc.edu/**
- **Washington:** Community Health Library (Kittitas Valley Community Hospital), **http://www.kvch.com/**
- **Washington:** Southwest Washington Medical Center Library (Southwest Washington Medical Center, Vancouver), **http://www.swmedicalcenter.com/body.cfm?id=72**

ONLINE GLOSSARIES

The Internet provides access to a number of free-to-use medical dictionaries. The National Library of Medicine has compiled the following list of online dictionaries:

- ADAM Medical Encyclopedia (A.D.A.M., Inc.), comprehensive medical reference: **http://www.nlm.nih.gov/medlineplus/encyclopedia.html**
- MedicineNet.com Medical Dictionary (MedicineNet, Inc.): **http://www.medterms.com/Script/Main/hp.asp**
- Merriam-Webster Medical Dictionary (Inteli-Health, Inc.): **http://www.intelihealth.com/IH/**
- Multilingual Glossary of Technical and Popular Medical Terms in Eight European Languages (European Commission) - Danish, Dutch, English, French, German, Italian, Portuguese, and Spanish: **http://allserv.rug.ac.be/~rvdstich/eugloss/welcome.html**
- On-line Medical Dictionary (CancerWEB): **http://cancerweb.ncl.ac.uk/omd/**
- Rare Diseases Terms (Office of Rare Diseases): **http://ord.aspensys.com/asp/diseases/diseases.asp**
- Technology Glossary (National Library of Medicine) - Health Care Technology: **http://www.nlm.nih.gov/nichsr/ta101/ta10108.htm**

Beyond these, MEDLINEplus contains a very patient-friendly encyclopedia covering every aspect of medicine (licensed from A.D.A.M., Inc.). The ADAM Medical Encyclopedia can be accessed at **http://www.nlm.nih.gov/medlineplus/encyclopedia.html**. ADAM is also available on commercial Web sites such as drkoop.com (**http://www.drkoop.com/**) and Web MD (**http://my.webmd.com/adam/asset/adam_disease_articles/a_to_z/a**). The NIH suggests the following Web sites in the ADAM Medical Encyclopedia when searching for information on polycystic ovarian syndrome:

- **Basic Guidelines for Polycystic Ovarian Syndrome**

    Stein-Leventhal syndrome
    Web site: http://www.nlm.nih.gov/medlineplus/ency/article/000369.htm

- **Signs & Symptoms for Polycystic Ovarian Syndrome**

    Amenorrhea
    Web site: http://www.nlm.nih.gov/medlineplus/ency/article/003149.htm

    Hirsutism
    Web site: http://www.nlm.nih.gov/medlineplus/ency/article/003148.htm

    Obese
    Web site: http://www.nlm.nih.gov/medlineplus/ency/article/003101.htm

    Obesity
    Web site: http://www.nlm.nih.gov/medlineplus/ency/article/003101.htm

- **Diagnostics and Tests for Polycystic Ovarian Syndrome**

    Biopsy
    Web site: http://www.nlm.nih.gov/medlineplus/ency/article/003416.htm

    Cysts
    Web site: http://www.nlm.nih.gov/medlineplus/ency/article/003240.htm

    Follicle-stimulating hormone
    Web site: http://www.nlm.nih.gov/medlineplus/ency/article/003710.htm

    FSH
    Web site: http://www.nlm.nih.gov/medlineplus/ency/article/003710.htm

    Laparoscopy
    Web site: http://www.nlm.nih.gov/medlineplus/ency/article/003918.htm

    LH
    Web site: http://www.nlm.nih.gov/medlineplus/ency/article/003708.htm

    Pregnancy test
    Web site: http://www.nlm.nih.gov/medlineplus/ency/article/003432.htm

    Serum HCG
    Web site: http://www.nlm.nih.gov/medlineplus/ency/article/003509.htm

    Testosterone
    Web site: http://www.nlm.nih.gov/medlineplus/ency/article/003707.htm

- **Background Topics for Polycystic Ovarian Syndrome**

    Virilization
    Web site: http://www.nlm.nih.gov/medlineplus/ency/article/002339.htm

    Weight reduction
    Web site: http://www.nlm.nih.gov/medlineplus/ency/article/001940.htm

Online Dictionary Directories

The following are additional online directories compiled by the National Library of Medicine, including a number of specialized medical dictionaries:

- Medical Dictionaries: Medical & Biological (World Health Organization):
  http://www.who.int/hlt/virtuallibrary/English/diction.htm#Medical

- MEL-Michigan Electronic Library List of Online Health and Medical Dictionaries (Michigan Electronic Library): **http://mel.lib.mi.us/health/health-dictionaries.html**

- Patient Education: Glossaries (DMOZ Open Directory Project):
  http://dmoz.org/Health/Education/Patient_Education/Glossaries/

- Web of Online Dictionaries (Bucknell University):
  http://www.yourdictionary.com/diction5.html#medicine

POLYCYSTIC OVARIAN SYNDROME DICTIONARY

The definitions below are derived from official public sources, including the National Institutes of Health [NIH] and the European Union [EU].

Abdomen: That portion of the body that lies between the thorax and the pelvis. [NIH]

Abdominal: Having to do with the abdomen, which is the part of the body between the chest and the hips that contains the pancreas, stomach, intestines, liver, gallbladder, and other organs. [NIH]

Aberrant: Wandering or deviating from the usual or normal course. [EU]

Ablation: The removal of an organ by surgery. [NIH]

Abortion: 1. The premature expulsion from the uterus of the products of conception - of the embryo, or of a nonviable fetus. The four classic symptoms, usually present in each type of abortion, are uterine contractions, uterine haemorrhage, softening and dilatation of the cervix, and presentation or expulsion of all or part of the products of conception. 2. Premature stoppage of a natural or a pathological process. [EU]

Acanthosis Nigricans: A circumscribed melanosis consisting of a brown-pigmented, velvety verrucosity or fine papillomatosis appearing in the axillae and other body folds. It occurs in association with endocrine disorders, underlying malignancy, administration of certain drugs, or as in inherited disorder. [NIH]

Acetylcholine: A neurotransmitter. Acetylcholine in vertebrates is the major transmitter at neuromuscular junctions, autonomic ganglia, parasympathetic effector junctions, a subset of sympathetic effector junctions, and at many sites in the central nervous system. It is generally not used as an administered drug because it is broken down very rapidly by cholinesterases, but it is useful in some ophthalmological applications. [NIH]

Acne: A disorder of the skin marked by inflammation of oil glands and hair glands. [NIH]

Acrylonitrile: A highly poisonous compound used widely in the manufacture of plastics, adhesives and synthetic rubber. [NIH]

Adaptability: Ability to develop some form of tolerance to conditions extremely different from those under which a living organism evolved. [NIH]

Adenovirus: A group of viruses that cause respiratory tract and eye infections. Adenoviruses used in gene therapy are altered to carry a specific tumor-fighting gene. [NIH]

Adhesions: Pathological processes consisting of the union of the opposing surfaces of a wound. [NIH]

Adhesives: Substances that cause the adherence of two surfaces. They include glues (properly collagen-derived adhesives), mucilages, sticky pastes, gums, resins, or latex. [NIH]

Adipocytes: Fat-storing cells found mostly in the abdominal cavity and subcutaneous tissue. Fat is usually stored in the form of tryglycerides. [NIH]

Adipose Tissue: Connective tissue composed of fat cells lodged in the meshes of areolar tissue. [NIH]

Adjuvant: A substance which aids another, such as an auxiliary remedy; in immunology, nonspecific stimulator (e.g., BCG vaccine) of the immune response. [EU]

Adolescence: The period of life beginning with the appearance of secondary sex characteristics and terminating with the cessation of somatic growth. The years usually referred to as adolescence lie between 13 and 18 years of age. [NIH]

Adrenal Cortex: The outer layer of the adrenal gland. It secretes mineralocorticoids, androgens, and glucocorticoids. [NIH]

Adrenal Glands: Paired glands situated in the retroperitoneal tissues at the superior pole of each kidney. [NIH]

Adrenal Medulla: The inner part of the adrenal gland; it synthesizes, stores and releases catecholamines. [NIH]

Adrenergic: Activated by, characteristic of, or secreting epinephrine or substances with similar activity; the term is applied to those nerve fibres that liberate norepinephrine at a synapse when a nerve impulse passes, i.e., the sympathetic fibres. [EU]

Adverse Effect: An unwanted side effect of treatment. [NIH]

Aerosol: A solution of a drug which can be atomized into a fine mist for inhalation therapy. [EU]

Afferent: Concerned with the transmission of neural impulse toward the central part of the nervous system. [NIH]

Affinity: 1. Inherent likeness or relationship. 2. A special attraction for a specific element, organ, or structure. 3. Chemical affinity; the force that binds atoms in molecules; the tendency of substances to combine by chemical reaction. 4. The strength of noncovalent chemical binding between two substances as measured by the dissociation constant of the complex. 5. In immunology, a thermodynamic expression of the strength of interaction between a single antigen-binding site and a single antigenic determinant (and thus of the stereochemical compatibility between them), most accurately applied to interactions among simple, uniform antigenic determinants such as haptens. Expressed as the association constant (K litres mole -1), which, owing to the heterogeneity of affinities in a population of antibody molecules of a given specificity, actually represents an average value (mean intrinsic association constant). 6. The reciprocal of the dissociation constant. [EU]

Agar: A complex sulfated polymer of galactose units, extracted from Gelidium cartilagineum, Gracilaria confervoides, and related red algae. It is used as a gel in the preparation of solid culture media for microorganisms, as a bulk laxative, in making emulsions, and as a supporting medium for immunodiffusion and immunoelectrophoresis. [NIH]

Age of Onset: The age or period of life at which a disease or the initial symptoms or manifestations of a disease appear in an individual. [NIH]

Agonist: In anatomy, a prime mover. In pharmacology, a drug that has affinity for and stimulates physiologic activity at cell receptors normally stimulated by naturally occurring substances. [EU]

Algorithms: A procedure consisting of a sequence of algebraic formulas and/or logical steps to calculate or determine a given task. [NIH]

Alkaline: Having the reactions of an alkali. [EU]

Alleles: Mutually exclusive forms of the same gene, occupying the same locus on homologous chromosomes, and governing the same biochemical and developmental process. [NIH]

Allergen: An antigenic substance capable of producing immediate-type hypersensitivity (allergy). [EU]

Alternative medicine: Practices not generally recognized by the medical community as standard or conventional medical approaches and used instead of standard treatments. Alternative medicine includes the taking of dietary supplements, megadose vitamins, and herbal preparations; the drinking of special teas; and practices such as massage therapy, magnet therapy, spiritual healing, and meditation. [NIH]

Alveoli: Tiny air sacs at the end of the bronchioles in the lungs. [NIH]

Amenorrhea: Absence of menstruation. [NIH]

Amino acid: Any organic compound containing an amino (-NH2 and a carboxyl (- COOH) group. The 20 a-amino acids listed in the accompanying table are the amino acids from which proteins are synthesized by formation of peptide bonds during ribosomal translation of messenger RNA; all except glycine, which is not optically active, have the L configuration. Other amino acids occurring in proteins, such as hydroxyproline in collagen, are formed by posttranslational enzymatic modification of amino acids residues in polypeptide chains. There are also several important amino acids, such as the neurotransmitter y-aminobutyric acid, that have no relation to proteins. Abbreviated AA. [EU]

Amino Acid Sequence: The order of amino acids as they occur in a polypeptide chain. This is referred to as the primary structure of proteins. It is of fundamental importance in determining protein conformation. [NIH]

Amplification: The production of additional copies of a chromosomal DNA sequence, found as either intrachromosomal or extrachromosomal DNA. [NIH]

Anabolic: Relating to, characterized by, or promoting anabolism. [EU]

Anaesthesia: Loss of feeling or sensation. Although the term is used for loss of tactile sensibility, or of any of the other senses, it is applied especially to loss of the sensation of pain, as it is induced to permit performance of surgery or other painful procedures. [EU]

Analog: In chemistry, a substance that is similar, but not identical, to another. [NIH]

Analogous: Resembling or similar in some respects, as in function or appearance, but not in origin or development;. [EU]

Anatomical: Pertaining to anatomy, or to the structure of the organism. [EU]

Androgen suppression: Treatment to suppress or block the production of male hormones. Androgen suppression is achieved by surgical removal of the testicles, by taking female sex hormones, or by taking other drugs. Also called androgen ablation. [NIH]

Androgen-Binding Protein: Carrier proteins produced in the Sertoli cells of the testis, secreted into the seminiferous tubules, and transported via the efferent ducts to the epididymis. They participate in the transport of androgens. Androgen-binding protein has the same amino acid sequence as sex hormone binding-globulin. They differ by their sites of synthesis and post-translational oligosacaccharide modifications. [NIH]

Androgenic: Producing masculine characteristics. [EU]

Androgens: A class of sex hormones associated with the development and maintenance of the secondary male sex characteristics, sperm induction, and sexual differentiation. In addition to increasing virility and libido, they also increase nitrogen and water retention and stimulate skeletal growth. [NIH]

Androstenedione: A steroid with androgenic properties that is produced in the testis, ovary, and adrenal cortex. It is a precursor to testosterone and other androgenic hormones. [NIH]

Anemia: A reduction in the number of circulating erythrocytes or in the quantity of hemoglobin. [NIH]

Aneurysm: A sac formed by the dilatation of the wall of an artery, a vein, or the heart. [NIH]

Angiography: Radiography of blood vessels after injection of a contrast medium. [NIH]

Angiotensinogen: An alpha-globulin of which a fragment of 14 amino acids is converted by renin to angiotensin I, the inactive precursor of angiotensin II. It is a member of the serpin superfamily. [NIH]

Animal model: An animal with a disease either the same as or like a disease in humans. Animal models are used to study the development and progression of diseases and to test new treatments before they are given to humans. Animals with transplanted human cancers or other tissues are called xenograft models. [NIH]

Anovulation: Suspension or cessation of ovulation in animals and humans. [NIH]

Antibacterial: A substance that destroys bacteria or suppresses their growth or reproduction. [EU]

Antibiotic: A drug used to treat infections caused by bacteria and other microorganisms. [NIH]

Antibody: A type of protein made by certain white blood cells in response to a foreign substance (antigen). Each antibody can bind to only a specific antigen. The purpose of this binding is to help destroy the antigen. Antibodies can work in several ways, depending on the nature of the antigen. Some antibodies destroy antigens directly. Others make it easier for white blood cells to destroy the antigen. [NIH]

Anticoagulant: A drug that helps prevent blood clots from forming. Also called a blood thinner. [NIH]

Anticonvulsant: An agent that prevents or relieves convulsions. [EU]

Antiemetic: An agent that prevents or alleviates nausea and vomiting. Also antinauseant. [EU]

Antiepileptic: An agent that combats epilepsy. [EU]

Antifungal: Destructive to fungi, or suppressing their reproduction or growth; effective against fungal infections. [EU]

Antigen: Any substance which is capable, under appropriate conditions, of inducing a specific immune response and of reacting with the products of that response, that is, with specific antibody or specifically sensitized T-lymphocytes, or both. Antigens may be soluble substances, such as toxins and foreign proteins, or particulate, such as bacteria and tissue cells; however, only the portion of the protein or polysaccharide molecule known as the antigenic determinant (q.v.) combines with antibody or a specific receptor on a lymphocyte. Abbreviated Ag. [EU]

Anti-inflammatory: Having to do with reducing inflammation. [NIH]

Anti-Inflammatory Agents: Substances that reduce or suppress inflammation. [NIH]

Antineoplastic: Inhibiting or preventing the development of neoplasms, checking the maturation and proliferation of malignant cells. [EU]

Anus: The opening of the rectum to the outside of the body. [NIH]

Apolipoproteins: The protein components of lipoproteins which remain after the lipids to which the proteins are bound have been removed. They play an important role in lipid transport and metabolism. [NIH]

Apoptosis: One of the two mechanisms by which cell death occurs (the other being the pathological process of necrosis). Apoptosis is the mechanism responsible for the physiological deletion of cells and appears to be intrinsically programmed. It is characterized by distinctive morphologic changes in the nucleus and cytoplasm, chromatin cleavage at regularly spaced sites, and the endonucleolytic cleavage of genomic DNA (DNA fragmentation) at internucleosomal sites. This mode of cell death serves as a balance to mitosis in regulating the size of animal tissues and in mediating pathologic processes associated with tumor growth. [NIH]

Arachidonic Acid: An unsaturated, essential fatty acid. It is found in animal and human fat as well as in the liver, brain, and glandular organs, and is a constituent of animal phosphatides. It is formed by the synthesis from dietary linoleic acid and is a precursor in the biosynthesis of prostaglandins, thromboxanes, and leukotrienes. [NIH]

Arterial: Pertaining to an artery or to the arteries. [EU]

Arteries: The vessels carrying blood away from the heart. [NIH]

Arteriolar: Pertaining to or resembling arterioles. [EU]

Arteriosclerosis: Thickening and loss of elasticity of arterial walls. Atherosclerosis is the most common form of arteriosclerosis and involves lipid deposition and thickening of the intimal cell layers within arteries. Additional forms of arteriosclerosis involve calcification of the media of muscular arteries (Monkeberg medial calcific sclerosis) and thickening of the walls of small arteries or arterioles due to cell proliferation or hyaline deposition (arteriolosclerosis). [NIH]

Artery: Vessel-carrying blood from the heart to various parts of the body. [NIH]

Arthrosis: A disease of a joint. [EU]

Assay: Determination of the amount of a particular constituent of a mixture, or of the biological or pharmacological potency of a drug. [EU]

Asymptomatic: Having no signs or symptoms of disease. [NIH]

Ataxia: Impairment of the ability to perform smoothly coordinated voluntary movements. This condition may affect the limbs, trunk, eyes, pharnyx, larnyx, and other structures. Ataxia may result from impaired sensory or motor function. Sensory ataxia may result from posterior column injury or peripheral nerve diseases. Motor ataxia may be associated with cerebellar diseases; cerebral cortex diseases; thalamic diseases; basal ganglia diseases; injury to the red nucleus; and other conditions. [NIH]

Atresia: Lack of a normal opening from the esophagus, intestines, or anus. [NIH]

Atrial: Pertaining to an atrium. [EU]

Atrioventricular: Pertaining to an atrium of the heart and to a ventricle. [EU]

Atrium: A chamber; used in anatomical nomenclature to designate a chamber affording entrance to another structure or organ. Usually used alone to designate an atrium of the heart. [EU]

Atrophy: Decrease in the size of a cell, tissue, organ, or multiple organs, associated with a variety of pathological conditions such as abnormal cellular changes, ischemia, malnutrition, or hormonal changes. [NIH]

Axillary: Pertaining to the armpit area, including the lymph nodes that are located there. [NIH]

Axillary Artery: The continuation of the subclavian artery; it distributes over the upper limb, axilla, chest and shoulder. [NIH]

Bacteria: Unicellular prokaryotic microorganisms which generally possess rigid cell walls, multiply by cell division, and exhibit three principal forms: round or coccal, rodlike or bacillary, and spiral or spirochetal. [NIH]

Bacteriophage: A virus whose host is a bacterial cell; A virus that exclusively infects bacteria. It generally has a protein coat surrounding the genome (DNA or RNA). One of the coliphages most extensively studied is the lambda phage, which is also one of the most important. [NIH]

Bacterium: Microscopic organism which may have a spherical, rod-like, or spiral unicellular or non-cellular body. Bacteria usually reproduce through asexual processes. [NIH]

Basal Ganglia: Large subcortical nuclear masses derived from the telencephalon and located in the basal regions of the cerebral hemispheres. [NIH]

Basal Ganglia Diseases: Diseases of the basal ganglia including the putamen; globus pallidus; claustrum; amygdala; and caudate nucleus. Dyskinesias (most notably involuntary movements and alterations of the rate of movement) represent the primary clinical manifestations of these disorders. Common etiologies include cerebrovascular disease; neurodegenerative diseases; and craniocerebral trauma. [NIH]

Base: In chemistry, the nonacid part of a salt; a substance that combines with acids to form salts; a substance that dissociates to give hydroxide ions in aqueous solutions; a substance whose molecule or ion can combine with a proton (hydrogen ion); a substance capable of donating a pair of electrons (to an acid) for the formation of a coordinate covalent bond. [EU]

Benign: Not cancerous; does not invade nearby tissue or spread to other parts of the body. [NIH]

Beta-Endorphin: A peptide consisting of amino acid sequence 61-91 of the endogenous pituitary hormone beta-lipotropin. The first four amino acids show a common tetrapeptide sequence with methionine- and leucine enkephalin. The compound shows opiate-like activity. Injection of beta-endorphin induces a profound analgesia of the whole body for several hours. This action is reversed after administration of naloxone. [NIH]

Bilateral: Affecting both the right and left side of body. [NIH]

Bile: An emulsifying agent produced in the liver and secreted into the duodenum. Its composition includes bile acids and salts, cholesterol, and electrolytes. It aids digestion of fats in the duodenum. [NIH]

Biochemical: Relating to biochemistry; characterized by, produced by, or involving chemical reactions in living organisms. [EU]

Biomarkers: Substances sometimes found in an increased amount in the blood, other body fluids, or tissues and that may suggest the presence of some types of cancer. Biomarkers include CA 125 (ovarian cancer), CA 15-3 (breast cancer), CEA (ovarian, lung, breast, pancreas, and GI tract cancers), and PSA (prostate cancer). Also called tumor markers. [NIH]

Biotechnology: Body of knowledge related to the use of organisms, cells or cell-derived constituents for the purpose of developing products which are technically, scientifically and clinically useful. Alteration of biologic function at the molecular level (i.e., genetic engineering) is a central focus; laboratory methods used include transfection and cloning technologies, sequence and structure analysis algorithms, computer databases, and gene and protein structure function analysis and prediction. [NIH]

Bipolar Disorder: A major affective disorder marked by severe mood swings (manic or major depressive episodes) and a tendency to remission and recurrence. [NIH]

Bladder: The organ that stores urine. [NIH]

Blastocyst: The mammalian embryo in the post-morula stage in which a fluid-filled cavity, enclosed primarily by trophoblast, contains an inner cell mass which becomes the embryonic disc. [NIH]

Blood Coagulation: The process of the interaction of blood coagulation factors that results in an insoluble fibrin clot. [NIH]

Blood Glucose: Glucose in blood. [NIH]

Blood pressure: The pressure of blood against the walls of a blood vessel or heart chamber. Unless there is reference to another location, such as the pulmonary artery or one of the heart chambers, it refers to the pressure in the systemic arteries, as measured, for example, in the forearm. [NIH]

Blood vessel: A tube in the body through which blood circulates. Blood vessels include a network of arteries, arterioles, capillaries, venules, and veins. [NIH]

Blot: To transfer DNA, RNA, or proteins to an immobilizing matrix such as nitrocellulose. [NIH]

Body Fluids: Liquid components of living organisms. [NIH]

Body Mass Index: One of the anthropometric measures of body mass; it has the highest correlation with skinfold thickness or body density. [NIH]

Bolus: A single dose of drug usually injected into a blood vessel over a short period of time. Also called bolus infusion. [NIH]

Bolus infusion: A single dose of drug usually injected into a blood vessel over a short period of time. Also called bolus. [NIH]

Bone Marrow: The soft tissue filling the cavities of bones. Bone marrow exists in two types, yellow and red. Yellow marrow is found in the large cavities of large bones and consists mostly of fat cells and a few primitive blood cells. Red marrow is a hematopoietic tissue and is the site of production of erythrocytes and granular leukocytes. Bone marrow is made up of a framework of connective tissue containing branching fibers with the frame being filled with marrow cells. [NIH]

Bowel: The long tube-shaped organ in the abdomen that completes the process of digestion. There is both a small and a large bowel. Also called the intestine. [NIH]

Bowel Movement: Body wastes passed through the rectum and anus. [NIH]

Brachial: All the nerves from the arm are ripped from the spinal cord. [NIH]

Brachial Artery: The continuation of the axillary artery; it branches into the radial and ulnar arteries. [NIH]

Branch: Most commonly used for branches of nerves, but applied also to other structures. [NIH]

Broad-spectrum: Effective against a wide range of microorganisms; said of an antibiotic. [EU]

Calcium: A basic element found in nearly all organized tissues. It is a member of the alkaline earth family of metals with the atomic symbol Ca, atomic number 20, and atomic weight 40. Calcium is the most abundant mineral in the body and combines with phosphorus to form calcium phosphate in the bones and teeth. It is essential for the normal functioning of nerves and muscles and plays a role in blood coagulation (as factor IV) and in many enzymatic processes. [NIH]

Calcium channel blocker: A drug used to relax the blood vessel and heart muscle, causing pressure inside blood vessels to drop. It also can regulate heart rhythm. [NIH]

Calcium Channel Blockers: A class of drugs that act by selective inhibition of calcium influx through cell membranes or on the release and binding of calcium in intracellular pools. Since they are inducers of vascular and other smooth muscle relaxation, they are used in the drug therapy of hypertension and cerebrovascular spasms, as myocardial protective agents, and in the relaxation of uterine spasms. [NIH]

Caloric intake: Refers to the number of calories (energy content) consumed. [NIH]

Carbamazepine: An anticonvulsant used to control grand mal and psychomotor or focal seizures. Its mode of action is not fully understood, but some of its actions resemble those of phenytoin; although there is little chemical resemblance between the two compounds, their three-dimensional structure is similar. [NIH]

Carbohydrate: An aldehyde or ketone derivative of a polyhydric alcohol, particularly of the pentahydric and hexahydric alcohols. They are so named because the hydrogen and oxygen are usually in the proportion to form water, (CH2O)n. The most important carbohydrates are the starches, sugars, celluloses, and gums. They are classified into mono-, di-, tri-, poly- and heterosaccharides. [EU]

Carbon Dioxide: A colorless, odorless gas that can be formed by the body and is necessary for the respiration cycle of plants and animals. [NIH]

Carcinogenic: Producing carcinoma. [EU]

Carcinogens: Substances that increase the risk of neoplasms in humans or animals. Both genotoxic chemicals, which affect DNA directly, and nongenotoxic chemicals, which induce neoplasms by other mechanism, are included. [NIH]

Carcinoma: Cancer that begins in the skin or in tissues that line or cover internal organs. [NIH]

Cardiac: Having to do with the heart. [NIH]

Cardiovascular: Having to do with the heart and blood vessels. [NIH]

Cardiovascular disease: Any abnormal condition characterized by dysfunction of the heart and blood vessels. CVD includes atherosclerosis (especially coronary heart disease, which can lead to heart attacks), cerebrovascular disease (e.g., stroke), and hypertension (high blood pressure). [NIH]

Carotene: The general name for a group of pigments found in green, yellow, and leafy vegetables, and yellow fruits. The pigments are fat-soluble, unsaturated aliphatic hydrocarbons functioning as provitamins and are converted to vitamin A through enzymatic processes in the intestinal wall. [NIH]

Case report: A detailed report of the diagnosis, treatment, and follow-up of an individual patient. Case reports also contain some demographic information about the patient (for example, age, gender, ethnic origin). [NIH]

Caspase: Enzyme released by the cell at a crucial stage in apoptosis in order to shred all cellular proteins. [NIH]

Castration: Surgical removal or artificial destruction of gonads. [NIH]

Catecholamine: A group of chemical substances manufactured by the adrenal medulla and secreted during physiological stress. [NIH]

Caudal: Denoting a position more toward the cauda, or tail, than some specified point of reference; same as inferior, in human anatomy. [EU]

Causal: Pertaining to a cause; directed against a cause. [EU]

Caveolins: The main structural proteins of caveolae. Several distinct genes for caveolins have been identified. [NIH]

Cell: The individual unit that makes up all of the tissues of the body. All living things are made up of one or more cells. [NIH]

Cell Aggregation: The phenomenon by which dissociated cells intermixed in vitro tend to group themselves with cells of their own type. [NIH]

Cell Death: The termination of the cell's ability to carry out vital functions such as metabolism, growth, reproduction, responsiveness, and adaptability. [NIH]

Cell Differentiation: Progressive restriction of the developmental potential and increasing specialization of function which takes place during the development of the embryo and leads to the formation of specialized cells, tissues, and organs. [NIH]

Cell Division: The fission of a cell. [NIH]

Cell membrane: Cell membrane = plasma membrane. The structure enveloping a cell, enclosing the cytoplasm, and forming a selective permeability barrier; it consists of lipids, proteins, and some carbohydrates, the lipids thought to form a bilayer in which integral proteins are embedded to varying degrees. [EU]

Cell proliferation: An increase in the number of cells as a result of cell growth and cell division. [NIH]

Cell Survival: The span of viability of a cell characterized by the capacity to perform certain functions such as metabolism, growth, reproduction, some form of responsiveness, and adaptability. [NIH]

Cerebellar: Pertaining to the cerebellum. [EU]

Cerebral: Of or pertaining of the cerebrum or the brain. [EU]

Cerebral Cortex: The thin layer of gray matter on the surface of the cerebral hemisphere that develops from the telencephalon and folds into gyri. It reaches its highest development in man and is responsible for intellectual faculties and higher mental functions. [NIH]

Cerebrovascular: Pertaining to the blood vessels of the cerebrum, or brain. [EU]

Cerebrum: The largest part of the brain. It is divided into two hemispheres, or halves, called the cerebral hemispheres. The cerebrum controls muscle functions of the body and also controls speech, emotions, reading, writing, and learning. [NIH]

Cervical: Relating to the neck, or to the neck of any organ or structure. Cervical lymph nodes are located in the neck; cervical cancer refers to cancer of the uterine cervix, which is the lower, narrow end (the "neck") of the uterus. [NIH]

Cervix: The lower, narrow end of the uterus that forms a canal between the uterus and vagina. [NIH]

Chemotaxis: The movement of cells or organisms toward or away from a substance in response to its concentration gradient. [NIH]

Chin: The anatomical frontal portion of the mandible, also known as the mentum, that contains the line of fusion of the two separate halves of the mandible (symphysis menti). This line of fusion divides inferiorly to enclose a triangular area called the mental protuberance. On each side, inferior to the second premolar tooth, is the mental foramen for the passage of blood vessels and a nerve. [NIH]

Cholesterol: The principal sterol of all higher animals, distributed in body tissues, especially the brain and spinal cord, and in animal fats and oils. [NIH]

Cholesterol Esters: Fatty acid esters of cholesterol which constitute about two-thirds of the cholesterol in the plasma. The accumulation of cholesterol esters in the arterial intima is a characteristic feature of atherosclerosis. [NIH]

Chromaffin System: The cells of the body which stain with chromium salts. They occur along the sympathetic nerves, in the adrenal gland, and in various other organs. [NIH]

Chromatin: The material of chromosomes. It is a complex of DNA, histones, and nonhistone proteins (chromosomal proteins, non-histone) found within the nucleus of a cell. [NIH]

Chromium: A trace element that plays a role in glucose metabolism. It has the atomic symbol Cr, atomic number 24, and atomic weight 52. According to the Fourth Annual Report on Carcinogens (NTP85-002,1985), chromium and some of its compounds have been listed as known carcinogens. [NIH]

Chromosomal: Pertaining to chromosomes. [EU]

Chromosome: Part of a cell that contains genetic information. Except for sperm and eggs, all human cells contain 46 chromosomes. [NIH]

Chronic: A disease or condition that persists or progresses over a long period of time. [NIH]

Chronic Disease: Disease or ailment of long duration. [NIH]

Chronic renal: Slow and progressive loss of kidney function over several years, often resulting in end-stage renal disease. People with end-stage renal disease need dialysis or transplantation to replace the work of the kidneys. [NIH]

Chylomicrons: A class of lipoproteins that carry dietary cholesterol and triglycerides from the small intestines to the tissues. [NIH]

Circulatory system: The system that contains the heart and the blood vessels and moves blood throughout the body. This system helps tissues get enough oxygen and nutrients, and it helps them get rid of waste products. The lymph system, which connects with the blood system, is often considered part of the circulatory system. [NIH]

CIS: Cancer Information Service. The CIS is the National Cancer Institute's link to the public, interpreting and explaining research findings in a clear and understandable manner, and providing personalized responses to specific questions about cancer. Access the CIS by calling 1-800-4-CANCER, or by using the Web site at http://cis.nci.nih.gov. [NIH]

Clamp: A u-shaped steel rod used with a pin or wire for skeletal traction in the treatment of certain fractures. [NIH]

Clathrin: The main structural coat protein of coated vesicles which play a key role in the intracellular transport between membranous organelles. Clathrin also interacts with cytoskeletal proteins. [NIH]

Clathrin-Coated Vesicles: Vesicles formed when cell-membrane coated pits invaginate and pinch off. The outer surface of these vesicles is covered with a lattice-like network of the protein dathrin. Shortly after formation, however, the clathrin coat is removed and the vesicles are referred to as endosomes. [NIH]

Clinical trial: A research study that tests how well new medical treatments or other interventions work in people. Each study is designed to test new methods of screening, prevention, diagnosis, or treatment of a disease. [NIH]

Clomiphene: A stilbene derivative that functions both as a partial estrogen agonist and complete estrogen antagonist depending on the target tissue. It antagonizes the estrogen receptor thereby initiating or augmenting ovulation in anovulatory women. [NIH]

Clone: The term "clone" has acquired a new meaning. It is applied specifically to the bits of inserted foreign DNA in the hybrid molecules of the population. Each inserted segment originally resided in the DNA of a complex genome amid millions of other DNA segment. [NIH]

Cloning: The production of a number of genetically identical individuals; in genetic engineering, a process for the efficient replication of a great number of identical DNA molecules. [NIH]

Coated Vesicles: Vesicles formed when cell-membrane coated pits invaginate and pinch off. The outer surface of these vesicles are covered with a lattice-like network of coat proteins, such as clathrin, coat protein complex proteins, or caveolins. [NIH]

Cofactor: A substance, microorganism or environmental factor that activates or enhances the action of another entity such as a disease-causing agent. [NIH]

Colon: The long, coiled, tubelike organ that removes water from digested food. The remaining material, solid waste called stool, moves through the colon to the rectum and leaves the body through the anus. [NIH]

Competency: The capacity of the bacterium to take up DNA from its surroundings. [NIH]

Complement: A term originally used to refer to the heat-labile factor in serum that causes immune cytolysis, the lysis of antibody-coated cells, and now referring to the entire functionally related system comprising at least 20 distinct serum proteins that is the effector not only of immune cytolysis but also of other biologic functions. Complement activation occurs by two different sequences, the classic and alternative pathways. The proteins of the classic pathway are termed 'components of complement' and are designated by the symbols C1 through C9. C1 is a calcium-dependent complex of three distinct proteins C1q, C1r and C1s. The proteins of the alternative pathway (collectively referred to as the properdin system) and complement regulatory proteins are known by semisystematic or trivial names. Fragments resulting from proteolytic cleavage of complement proteins are designated with lower-case letter suffixes, e.g., C3a. Inactivated fragments may be designated with the suffix 'i', e.g. C3bi. Activated components or complexes with biological activity are designated by a bar over the symbol e.g. C1 or C4b,2a. The classic pathway is activated by the binding of C1 to classic pathway activators, primarily antigen-antibody complexes containing IgM, IgG1, IgG3; C1q binds to a single IgM molecule or two adjacent IgG molecules. The alternative pathway can be activated by IgA immune complexes and also by nonimmunologic materials including bacterial endotoxins, microbial polysaccharides, and cell walls. Activation of the classic pathway triggers an enzymatic cascade involving C1, C4, C2 and C3; activation of the alternative pathway triggers a cascade involving C3 and factors B, D and P. Both result in the cleavage of C5 and the formation of the membrane attack complex. Complement activation also results in the formation of many biologically active complement fragments that act as anaphylatoxins, opsonins, or chemotactic factors. [EU]

Complementary and alternative medicine: CAM. Forms of treatment that are used in addition to (complementary) or instead of (alternative) standard treatments. These practices are not considered standard medical approaches. CAM includes dietary supplements, megadose vitamins, herbal preparations, special teas, massage therapy, magnet therapy, spiritual healing, and meditation. [NIH]

Complementary medicine: Practices not generally recognized by the medical community as standard or conventional medical approaches and used to enhance or complement the standard treatments. Complementary medicine includes the taking of dietary supplements, megadose vitamins, and herbal preparations; the drinking of special teas; and practices such as massage therapy, magnet therapy, spiritual healing, and meditation. [NIH]

Compliance: Distensibility measure of a chamber such as the lungs (lung compliance) or bladder. Compliance is expressed as a change in volume per unit change in pressure. [NIH]

Computational Biology: A field of biology concerned with the development of techniques for the collection and manipulation of biological data, and the use of such data to make biological discoveries or predictions. This field encompasses all computational methods and theories applicable to molecular biology and areas of computer-based techniques for solving biological problems including manipulation of models and datasets. [NIH]

Computed tomography: CT scan. A series of detailed pictures of areas inside the body, taken from different angles; the pictures are created by a computer linked to an x-ray machine. Also called computerized tomography and computerized axial tomography (CAT) scan. [NIH]

Computerized tomography: A series of detailed pictures of areas inside the body, taken from different angles; the pictures are created by a computer linked to an x-ray machine. Also called computerized axial tomography (CAT) scan and computed tomography (CT scan). [NIH]

Conception: The onset of pregnancy, marked by implantation of the blastocyst; the formation of a viable zygote. [EU]

Cones: One type of specialized light-sensitive cells (photoreceptors) in the retina that provide sharp central vision and color vision. [NIH]

Conjugated: Acting or operating as if joined; simultaneous. [EU]

Connective Tissue: Tissue that supports and binds other tissues. It consists of connective tissue cells embedded in a large amount of extracellular matrix. [NIH]

Connective Tissue: Tissue that supports and binds other tissues. It consists of connective tissue cells embedded in a large amount of extracellular matrix. [NIH]

Connective Tissue Cells: A group of cells that includes fibroblasts, cartilage cells, adipocytes, smooth muscle cells, and bone cells. [NIH]

Contraception: Use of agents, devices, methods, or procedures which diminish the likelihood of or prevent conception. [NIH]

Contraceptive Agents: Chemical substances that prevent or reduce the probability of conception. [NIH]

Contraindications: Any factor or sign that it is unwise to pursue a certain kind of action or treatment, e. g. giving a general anesthetic to a person with pneumonia. [NIH]

Contrast medium: A substance that is introduced into or around a structure and, because of the difference in absorption of x-rays by the contrast medium and the surrounding tissues, allows radiographic visualization of the structure. [EU]

Control group: In a clinical trial, the group that does not receive the new treatment being studied. This group is compared to the group that receives the new treatment, to see if the new treatment works. [NIH]

Controlled study: An experiment or clinical trial that includes a comparison (control) group. [NIH]

Conventional therapy: A currently accepted and widely used treatment for a certain type of disease, based on the results of past research. Also called conventional treatment. [NIH]

Conventional treatment: A currently accepted and widely used treatment for a certain type of disease, based on the results of past research. Also called conventional therapy. [NIH]

Convulsions: A general term referring to sudden and often violent motor activity of cerebral or brainstem origin. Convulsions may also occur in the absence of an electrical cerebral discharge (e.g., in response to hypotension). [NIH]

Coordination: Muscular or motor regulation or the harmonious cooperation of muscles or groups of muscles, in a complex action or series of actions. [NIH]

Cor: The muscular organ that maintains the circulation of the blood. c. adiposum a heart that has undergone fatty degeneration or that has an accumulation of fat around it; called also fat or fatty, heart. c. arteriosum the left side of the heart, so called because it contains oxygenated (arterial) blood. c. biloculare a congenital anomaly characterized by failure of formation of the atrial and ventricular septums, the heart having only two chambers, a single atrium and a single ventricle, and a common atrioventricular valve. c. bovinum (L. 'ox heart') a greatly enlarged heart due to a hypertrophied left ventricle; called also c. taurinum and bucardia. c. dextrum (L. 'right heart') the right atrium and ventricle. c. hirsutum, c. villosum. c. mobile (obs.) an abnormally movable heart. c. pendulum a heart so movable that it seems to be hanging by the great blood vessels. c. pseudotriloculare biatriatum a congenital cardiac anomaly in which the heart functions as a three-chambered heart because of tricuspid atresia, the right ventricle being extremely small or rudimentary and the right atrium greatly dilated. Blood passes from the right to the left atrium and thence disease due to pulmonary hypertension secondary to disease of the lung, or its blood vessels, with hypertrophy of the right ventricle. [EU]

Cornea: The transparent part of the eye that covers the iris and the pupil and allows light to enter the inside. [NIH]

Coronary: Encircling in the manner of a crown; a term applied to vessels; nerves, ligaments, etc. The term usually denotes the arteries that supply the heart muscle and, by extension, a pathologic involvement of them. [EU]

Coronary heart disease: A type of heart disease caused by narrowing of the coronary arteries that feed the heart, which needs a constant supply of oxygen and nutrients carried by the blood in the coronary arteries. When the coronary arteries become narrowed or clogged by fat and cholesterol deposits and cannot supply enough blood to the heart, CHD results. [NIH]

Coronary Thrombosis: Presence of a thrombus in a coronary artery, often causing a myocardial infarction. [NIH]

Corpus: The body of the uterus. [NIH]

Corpus Luteum: The yellow glandular mass formed in the ovary by an ovarian follicle that has ruptured and discharged its ovum. [NIH]

Cortex: The outer layer of an organ or other body structure, as distinguished from the internal substance. [EU]

Cortical: Pertaining to or of the nature of a cortex or bark. [EU]

Corticosteroid: Any of the steroids elaborated by the adrenal cortex (excluding the sex hormones of adrenal origin) in response to the release of corticotrophin (adrenocorticotropic hormone) by the pituitary gland, to any of the synthetic equivalents of these steroids, or to angiotensin II. They are divided, according to their predominant biological activity, into three major groups: glucocorticoids, chiefly influencing carbohydrate, fat, and protein metabolism; mineralocorticoids, affecting the regulation of electrolyte and water balance; and C19 androgens. Some corticosteroids exhibit both types of activity in varying degrees, and others exert only one type of effect. The corticosteroids are used clinically for hormonal replacement therapy, for suppression of ACTH secretion by the anterior pituitary, as antineoplastic, antiallergic, and anti-inflammatory agents, and to suppress the immune response. Called also adrenocortical hormone and corticoid. [EU]

Corticotropin-Releasing Hormone: A neuropeptide released by the hypothalamus that stimulates the release of corticotropin by the anterior pituitary gland. [NIH]

Cortisol: A steroid hormone secreted by the adrenal cortex as part of the body's response to stress. [NIH]

Cortisone: A natural steroid hormone produced in the adrenal gland. It can also be made in the laboratory. Cortisone reduces swelling and can suppress immune responses. [NIH]

Cost-benefit: A quantitative technique of economic analysis which, when applied to radiation practice, compares the health detriment from the radiation doses concerned with the cost of radiation dose reduction in that practice. [NIH]

Cost-Benefit Analysis: A method of comparing the cost of a program with its expected benefits in dollars (or other currency). The benefit-to-cost ratio is a measure of total return expected per unit of money spent. This analysis generally excludes consideration of factors that are not measured ultimately in economic terms. Cost effectiveness compares alternative ways to achieve a specific set of results. [NIH]

Cyclic: Pertaining to or occurring in a cycle or cycles; the term is applied to chemical compounds that contain a ring of atoms in the nucleus. [EU]

Cyclin: Molecule that regulates the cell cycle. [NIH]

Cyclin-Dependent Kinases: Protein kinases that control cell cycle progression in all eukaryotes and require physical association with cyclins to achieve full enzymatic activity. Cyclin-dependent kinases are regulated by phosphorylation and dephosphorylation events. [NIH]

Cyproterone: An anti-androgen that, in the form of its acetate, also has progestational properties. It is used in the treatment of hypersexuality in males, as a palliative in prostatic carcinoma, and, in combination with estrogen, for the therapy of severe acne and hirsutism in females. [NIH]

Cyproterone Acetate: An agent with anti-androgen and progestational properties. It shows competitive binding with dihydrotestosterone at androgen receptor sites. [NIH]

Cyst: A sac or capsule filled with fluid. [NIH]

Cytochrome: Any electron transfer hemoprotein having a mode of action in which the transfer of a single electron is effected by a reversible valence change of the central iron atom of the heme prosthetic group between the +2 and +3 oxidation states; classified as cytochromes a in which the heme contains a formyl side chain, cytochromes b, which contain protoheme or a closely similar heme that is not covalently bound to the protein, cytochromes c in which protoheme or other heme is covalently bound to the protein, and cytochromes d in which the iron-tetrapyrrole has fewer conjugated double bonds than the hemes have. Well-known cytochromes have been numbered consecutively within groups and are designated by subscripts (beginning with no subscript), e.g. cytochromes c, c1, C2, . New cytochromes are named according to the wavelength in nanometres of the absorption maximum of the a-band of the iron (II) form in pyridine, e.g., c-555. [EU]

Cytoplasm: The protoplasm of a cell exclusive of that of the nucleus; it consists of a continuous aqueous solution (cytosol) and the organelles and inclusions suspended in it (phaneroplasm), and is the site of most of the chemical activities of the cell. [EU]

Cytotoxic: Cell-killing. [NIH]

Decidua: The epithelial lining of the endometrium that is formed before the fertilized ovum reaches the uterus. The fertilized ovum embeds in the decidua. If the ovum is not fertilized, the decidua is shed during menstruation. [NIH]

Dehydroepiandrosterone: DHEA. A substance that is being studied as a cancer prevention drug. It belongs to the family of drugs called steroids. [NIH]

Deletion: A genetic rearrangement through loss of segments of DNA (chromosomes), bringing sequences, which are normally separated, into close proximity. [NIH]

Dendrites: Extensions of the nerve cell body. They are short and branched and receive stimuli from other neurons. [NIH]

Density: The logarithm to the base 10 of the opacity of an exposed and processed film. [NIH]

Dentition: The teeth in the dental arch; ordinarily used to designate the natural teeth in position in their alveoli. [EU]

Deoxyribonucleic: A polymer of subunits called deoxyribonucleotides which is the primary genetic material of a cell, the material equivalent to genetic information. [NIH]

Deoxyribonucleic acid: A polymer of subunits called deoxyribonucleotides which is the primary genetic material of a cell, the material equivalent to genetic information. [NIH]

Depolarization: The process or act of neutralizing polarity. In neurophysiology, the reversal of the resting potential in excitable cell membranes when stimulated, i.e., the tendency of the cell membrane potential to become positive with respect to the potential outside the cell. [EU]

Depressive Disorder: An affective disorder manifested by either a dysphoric mood or loss of interest or pleasure in usual activities. The mood disturbance is prominent and relatively persistent. [NIH]

Desensitization: The prevention or reduction of immediate hypersensitivity reactions by administration of graded doses of allergen; called also hyposensitization and immunotherapy. [EU]

Dexamethasone: (11 beta,16 alpha)-9-Fluoro-11,17,21-trihydroxy-16-methylpregna-1,4-diene-3,20-dione. An anti-inflammatory glucocorticoid used either in the free alcohol or esterified form in treatment of conditions that respond generally to cortisone. [NIH]

Diabetes Insipidus: A metabolic disorder due to disorders in the production or release of vasopressin. It is characterized by the chronic excretion of large amounts of low specific gravity urine and great thirst. [NIH]

Diabetes Mellitus: A heterogeneous group of disorders that share glucose intolerance in common. [NIH]

Diabetic Ketoacidosis: Complication of diabetes resulting from severe insulin deficiency coupled with an absolute or relative increase in glucagon concentration. The metabolic acidosis is caused by the breakdown of adipose stores and resulting increased levels of free fatty acids. Glucagon accelerates the oxidation of the free fatty acids producing excess ketone bodies (ketosis). [NIH]

Diagnostic procedure: A method used to identify a disease. [NIH]

Diastolic: Of or pertaining to the diastole. [EU]

Diathermy: The induction of local hyperthermia by either short radio waves or high-frequency sound waves. [NIH]

Diencephalon: The paired caudal parts of the prosencephalon from which the thalamus, hypothalamus, epithalamus, and subthalamus are derived. [NIH]

Digestion: The process of breakdown of food for metabolism and use by the body. [NIH]

Digestive system: The organs that take in food and turn it into products that the body can use to stay healthy. Waste products the body cannot use leave the body through bowel movements. The digestive system includes the salivary glands, mouth, esophagus, stomach, liver, pancreas, gallbladder, small and large intestines, and rectum. [NIH]

Dihydrotestosterone: Anabolic agent. [NIH]

Dilatation: The act of dilating. [NIH]

Dilatation, Pathologic: The condition of an anatomical structure's being dilated beyond normal dimensions. [NIH]

Dilation: A process by which the pupil is temporarily enlarged with special eye drops (mydriatic); allows the eye care specialist to better view the inside of the eye. [NIH]

Dimerization: The process by which two molecules of the same chemical composition form a condensation product or polymer. [NIH]

Direct: 1. Straight; in a straight line. 2. Performed immediately and without the intervention of subsidiary means. [EU]

Discrete: Made up of separate parts or characterized by lesions which do not become blended; not running together; separate. [NIH]

Dissociation: 1. The act of separating or state of being separated. 2. The separation of a molecule into two or more fragments (atoms, molecules, ions, or free radicals) produced by the absorption of light or thermal energy or by solvation. 3. In psychology, a defense mechanism in which a group of mental processes are segregated from the rest of a person's mental activity in order to avoid emotional distress, as in the dissociative disorders (q.v.), or in which an idea or object is segregated from its emotional significance; in the first sense it is roughly equivalent to splitting, in the second, to isolation. 4. A defect of mental integration in which one or more groups of mental processes become separated off from normal consciousness and, thus separated, function as a unitary whole. [EU]

Domperidone: A specific blocker of dopamine receptors. It speeds gastrointestinal peristalsis, causes prolactin release, and is used as antiemetic and tool in the study of dopaminergic mechanisms. [NIH]

Dopa: The racemic or DL form of DOPA, an amino acid found in various legumes. The dextro form has little physiologic activity but the levo form (levodopa) is a very important physiologic mediator and precursor and pharmacological agent. [NIH]

Dopamine: An endogenous catecholamine and prominent neurotransmitter in several systems of the brain. In the synthesis of catecholamines from tyrosine, it is the immediate precursor to norepinephrine and epinephrine. Dopamine is a major transmitter in the extrapyramidal system of the brain, and important in regulating movement. A family of dopaminergic receptor subtypes mediate its action. Dopamine is used pharmacologically for its direct (beta adrenergic agonist) and indirect (adrenergic releasing) sympathomimetic effects including its actions as an inotropic agent and as a renal vasodilator. [NIH]

Dopamine Agonists: Drugs that bind to and activate dopamine receptors. [NIH]

Drive: A state of internal activity of an organism that is a necessary condition before a given stimulus will elicit a class of responses; e.g., a certain level of hunger (drive) must be present before food will elicit an eating response. [NIH]

Dyslipidemia: Disorders in the lipoprotein metabolism; classified as hypercholesterolemia, hypertriglyceridemia, combined hyperlipidemia, and low levels of high-density lipoprotein (HDL) cholesterol. All of the dyslipidemias can be primary or secondary. Both elevated levels of low-density lipoprotein (LDL) cholesterol and low levels of HDL cholesterol predispose to premature atherosclerosis. [NIH]

Dysphoric: A feeling of unpleasantness and discomfort. [NIH]

Dysplasia: Cells that look abnormal under a microscope but are not cancer. [NIH]

Dystrophy: Any disorder arising from defective or faulty nutrition, especially the muscular dystrophies. [EU]

Eclampsia: Onset of convulsions or coma in a previously diagnosed pre-eclamptic patient. [NIH]

Edema: Excessive amount of watery fluid accumulated in the intercellular spaces, most commonly present in subcutaneous tissue. [NIH]

Effector: It is often an enzyme that converts an inactive precursor molecule into an active second messenger. [NIH]

Efficacy: The extent to which a specific intervention, procedure, regimen, or service produces a beneficial result under ideal conditions. Ideally, the determination of efficacy is based on the results of a randomized control trial. [NIH]

Elective: Subject to the choice or decision of the patient or physician; applied to procedures that are advantageous to the patient but not urgent. [EU]

Electrolyte: A substance that dissociates into ions when fused or in solution, and thus becomes capable of conducting electricity; an ionic solute. [EU]

Electrophysiological: Pertaining to electrophysiology, that is a branch of physiology that is concerned with the electric phenomena associated with living bodies and involved in their functional activity. [EU]

Embryo: The prenatal stage of mammalian development characterized by rapid morphological changes and the differentiation of basic structures. [NIH]

Embryo Transfer: Removal of a mammalian embryo from one environment and replacement in the same or a new environment. The embryo is usually in the pre-nidation phase, i.e., a blastocyst. The process includes embryo or blastocyst transplantation or transfer after in vitro fertilization and transfer of the inner cell mass of the blastocyst. It is not used for transfer of differentiated embryonic tissue, e.g., germ layer cells. [NIH]

Encapsulated: Confined to a specific, localized area and surrounded by a thin layer of tissue. [NIH]

Endocrine Glands: Ductless glands that secrete substances which are released directly into the circulation and which influence metabolism and other body functions. [NIH]

Endocrine System: The system of glands that release their secretions (hormones) directly into the circulatory system. In addition to the endocrine glands, included are the chromaffin system and the neurosecretory systems. [NIH]

Endocrinology: A subspecialty of internal medicine concerned with the metabolism, physiology, and disorders of the endocrine system. [NIH]

Endogenous: Produced inside an organism or cell. The opposite is external (exogenous) production. [NIH]

Endometrial: Having to do with the endometrium (the layer of tissue that lines the uterus). [NIH]

Endometriosis: A condition in which tissue more or less perfectly resembling the uterine mucous membrane (the endometrium) and containing typical endometrial granular and stromal elements occurs aberrantly in various locations in the pelvic cavity. [NIH]

Endometrium: The layer of tissue that lines the uterus. [NIH]

Endorphins: One of the three major groups of endogenous opioid peptides. They are large peptides derived from the pro-opiomelanocortin precursor. The known members of this group are alpha-, beta-, and gamma-endorphin. The term endorphin is also sometimes used to refer to all opioid peptides, but the narrower sense is used here; opioid peptides is used for the broader group. [NIH]

Endosomes: Cytoplasmic vesicles formed when coated vesicles shed their clathrin coat. Endosomes internalize macromolecules bound by receptors on the cell surface. [NIH]

End-stage renal: Total chronic kidney failure. When the kidneys fail, the body retains fluid and harmful wastes build up. A person with ESRD needs treatment to replace the work of the failed kidneys. [NIH]

Energy balance: Energy is the capacity of a body or a physical system for doing work. Energy balance is the state in which the total energy intake equals total energy needs. [NIH]

Enkephalin: A natural opiate painkiller, in the hypothalamus. [NIH]

Environmental Exposure: The exposure to potentially harmful chemical, physical, or biological agents in the environment or to environmental factors that may include ionizing radiation, pathogenic organisms, or toxic chemicals. [NIH]

Environmental Health: The science of controlling or modifying those conditions, influences, or forces surrounding man which relate to promoting, establishing, and maintaining health. [NIH]

Enzymatic: Phase where enzyme cuts the precursor protein. [NIH]

Enzyme: A protein that speeds up chemical reactions in the body. [NIH]

Enzyme-Linked Immunosorbent Assay: An immunoassay utilizing an antibody labeled with an enzyme marker such as horseradish peroxidase. While either the enzyme or the antibody is bound to an immunosorbent substrate, they both retain their biologic activity; the change in enzyme activity as a result of the enzyme-antibody-antigen reaction is proportional to the concentration of the antigen and can be measured spectrophotometrically or with the naked eye. Many variations of the method have been developed. [NIH]

Epinephrine: The active sympathomimetic hormone from the adrenal medulla in most species. It stimulates both the alpha- and beta- adrenergic systems, causes systemic vasoconstriction and gastrointestinal relaxation, stimulates the heart, and dilates bronchi and cerebral vessels. It is used in asthma and cardiac failure and to delay absorption of local anesthetics. [NIH]

Epithelial: Refers to the cells that line the internal and external surfaces of the body. [NIH]

Epithelial Cells: Cells that line the inner and outer surfaces of the body. [NIH]

Epithelium: One or more layers of epithelial cells, supported by the basal lamina, which covers the inner or outer surfaces of the body. [NIH]

Erythrocytes: Red blood cells. Mature erythrocytes are non-nucleated, biconcave disks containing hemoglobin whose function is to transport oxygen. [NIH]

Esophagus: The muscular tube through which food passes from the throat to the stomach. [NIH]

Essential Tremor: A rhythmic, involuntary, purposeless, oscillating movement resulting from the alternate contraction and relaxation of opposing groups of muscles. [NIH]

Estradiol: The most potent mammalian estrogenic hormone. It is produced in the ovary, placenta, testis, and possibly the adrenal cortex. [NIH]

Estrogen: One of the two female sex hormones. [NIH]

Estrogen receptor: ER. Protein found on some cancer cells to which estrogen will attach. [NIH]

Ethinyl Estradiol: A semisynthetic estrogen with high oral estrogenic potency. It is often used as the estrogenic component in oral contraceptives. [NIH]

Excitation: An act of irritation or stimulation or of responding to a stimulus; the addition of energy, as the excitation of a molecule by absorption of photons. [EU]

Exogenous: Developed or originating outside the organism, as exogenous disease. [EU]

Extrapyramidal: Outside of the pyramidal tracts. [EU]

Eye Infections: Infection, moderate to severe, caused by bacteria, fungi, or viruses, which occurs either on the external surface of the eye or intraocularly with probable inflammation, visual impairment, or blindness. [NIH]

Facial: Of or pertaining to the face. [EU]

Fallopian tube: The oviduct, a muscular tube about 10 cm long, lying in the upper border of the broad ligament. [NIH]

Family Planning: Programs or services designed to assist the family in controlling reproduction by either improving or diminishing fertility. [NIH]

Fat: Total lipids including phospholipids. [NIH]

Fatty acids: A major component of fats that are used by the body for energy and tissue development. [NIH]

Fertilization in Vitro: Fertilization of an egg outside the body when the egg is normally fertilized in the body. [NIH]

Fetus: The developing offspring from 7 to 8 weeks after conception until birth. [NIH]

Fibrin: A protein derived from fibrinogen in the presence of thrombin, which forms part of the blood clot. [NIH]

Fibrosis: Any pathological condition where fibrous connective tissue invades any organ, usually as a consequence of inflammation or other injury. [NIH]

Flutamide: An antiandrogen with about the same potency as cyproterone in rodent and canine species. [NIH]

Fold: A plication or doubling of various parts of the body. [NIH]

Follicles: Shafts through which hair grows. [NIH]

Follicular Fluid: A fluid consisting of sex steroid hormones, plasma proteins, mucopolysaccharides, and electrolytes that is present in the vesicular ovarian follicle (Graafian follicle) surrounding the ovum. [NIH]

Follicular Phase: The period of the menstrual cycle that begins with menstruation and ends with ovulation. [NIH]

Forearm: The part between the elbow and the wrist. [NIH]

Gallbladder: The pear-shaped organ that sits below the liver. Bile is concentrated and stored in the gallbladder. [NIH]

Ganglia: Clusters of multipolar neurons surrounded by a capsule of loosely organized connective tissue located outside the central nervous system. [NIH]

Gas: Air that comes from normal breakdown of food. The gases are passed out of the body through the rectum (flatus) or the mouth (burp). [NIH]

Gastrin: A hormone released after eating. Gastrin causes the stomach to produce more acid. [NIH]

Gastrointestinal: Refers to the stomach and intestines. [NIH]

Gastrointestinal tract: The stomach and intestines. [NIH]

Gene: The functional and physical unit of heredity passed from parent to offspring. Genes are pieces of DNA, and most genes contain the information for making a specific protein. [NIH]

Gene Expression: The phenotypic manifestation of a gene or genes by the processes of gene action. [NIH]

Gene Therapy: The introduction of new genes into cells for the purpose of treating disease by restoring or adding gene expression. Techniques include insertion of retroviral vectors, transfection, homologous recombination, and injection of new genes into the nuclei of single cell embryos. The entire gene therapy process may consist of multiple steps. The new genes may be introduced into proliferating cells in vivo (e.g., bone marrow) or in vitro (e.g., fibroblast cultures) and the modified cells transferred to the site where the gene expression is required. Gene therapy may be particularly useful for treating enzyme deficiency diseases, hemoglobinopathies, and leukemias and may also prove useful in restoring drug sensitivity, particularly for leukemia. [NIH]

Generator: Any system incorporating a fixed parent radionuclide from which is produced a daughter radionuclide which is to be removed by elution or by any other method and used in a radiopharmaceutical. [NIH]

Genotype: The genetic constitution of the individual; the characterization of the genes. [NIH]

Germ Cells: The reproductive cells in multicellular organisms. [NIH]

Gestation: The period of development of the young in viviparous animals, from the time of fertilization of the ovum until birth. [EU]

Gestational: Psychosis attributable to or occurring during pregnancy. [NIH]

Gland: An organ that produces and releases one or more substances for use in the body. Some glands produce fluids that affect tissues or organs. Others produce hormones or participate in blood production. [NIH]

Glucocorticoid: A compound that belongs to the family of compounds called corticosteroids (steroids). Glucocorticoids affect metabolism and have anti-inflammatory and immunosuppressive effects. They may be naturally produced (hormones) or synthetic (drugs). [NIH]

Gluconeogenesis: The process by which glucose is formed from a non-carbohydrate source. [NIH]

Glucose: D-Glucose. A primary source of energy for living organisms. It is naturally occurring and is found in fruits and other parts of plants in its free state. It is used therapeutically in fluid and nutrient replacement. [NIH]

Glucose Intolerance: A pathological state in which the fasting plasma glucose level is less than 140 mg per deciliter and the 30-, 60-, or 90-minute plasma glucose concentration following a glucose tolerance test exceeds 200 mg per deciliter. This condition is seen frequently in diabetes mellitus but also occurs with other diseases. [NIH]

Glucose tolerance: The power of the normal liver to absorb and store large quantities of glucose and the effectiveness of intestinal absorption of glucose. The glucose tolerance test is a metabolic test of carbohydrate tolerance that measures active insulin, a hepatic function based on the ability of the liver to absorb glucose. The test consists of ingesting 100 grams of glucose into a fasting stomach; blood sugar should return to normal in 2 to 21 hours after ingestion. [NIH]

Glucose Tolerance Test: Determination of whole blood or plasma sugar in a fasting state before and at prescribed intervals (usually 1/2 hr, 1 hr, 3 hr, 4 hr) after taking a specified amount (usually 100 gm orally) of glucose. [NIH]

Glutamic Acid: A non-essential amino acid naturally occurring in the L-form. Glutamic acid (glutamate) is the most common excitatory neurotransmitter in the central nervous system. [NIH]

Glycine: A non-essential amino acid. It is found primarily in gelatin and silk fibroin and used therapeutically as a nutrient. It is also a fast inhibitory neurotransmitter. [NIH]

Glycoprotein: A protein that has sugar molecules attached to it. [NIH]

Glycosuria: The presence of glucose in the urine, especially the excretion of an abnormally large amount of sugar (glucose) in the urine, i.e., more than 1 gm. in 24 hours. [EU]

Gonad: A sex organ, such as an ovary or a testicle, which produces the gametes in most multicellular animals. [NIH]

Gonadal: Pertaining to a gonad. [EU]

Gonadorelin: A decapeptide hormone released by the hypothalamus. It stimulates the synthesis and secretion of both follicle-stimulating hormone (FSH) and luteinizing hormone (LH) from the pituitary gland. [NIH]

Gonadotropic: Stimulating the gonads; applied to hormones of the anterior pituitary which influence the gonads. [EU]

Gonadotropin: The water-soluble follicle stimulating substance, by some believed to originate in chorionic tissue, obtained from the serum of pregnant mares. It is used to supplement the action of estrogens. [NIH]

Governing Board: The group in which legal authority is vested for the control of health-related institutions and organizations. [NIH]

Grade: The grade of a tumor depends on how abnormal the cancer cells look under a microscope and how quickly the tumor is likely to grow and spread. Grading systems are different for each type of cancer. [NIH]

Graft: Healthy skin, bone, or other tissue taken from one part of the body and used to replace diseased or injured tissue removed from another part of the body. [NIH]

Grafting: The operation of transfer of tissue from one site to another. [NIH]

Granulocytes: Leukocytes with abundant granules in the cytoplasm. They are divided into three groups: neutrophils, eosinophils, and basophils. [NIH]

Granulosa Cells: Cells of the membrana granulosa lining the vesicular ovarian follicle which become luteal cells after ovulation. [NIH]

Growth: The progressive development of a living being or part of an organism from its earliest stage to maturity. [NIH]

Haplotypes: The genetic constitution of individuals with respect to one member of a pair of allelic genes, or sets of genes that are closely linked and tend to be inherited together such as those of the major histocompatibility complex. [NIH]

Haptens: Small antigenic determinants capable of eliciting an immune response only when coupled to a carrier. Haptens bind to antibodies but by themselves cannot elicit an antibody response. [NIH]

Headache: Pain in the cranial region that may occur as an isolated and benign symptom or as a manifestation of a wide variety of conditions including subarachnoid hemorrhage; craniocerebral trauma; central nervous system infections; intracranial hypertension; and other disorders. In general, recurrent headaches that are not associated with a primary disease process are referred to as headache disorders (e.g., migraine). [NIH]

Heart attack: A seizure of weak or abnormal functioning of the heart. [NIH]

Heme: The color-furnishing portion of hemoglobin. It is found free in tissues and as the prosthetic group in many hemeproteins. [NIH]

Hemoglobin: One of the fractions of glycosylated hemoglobin A1c. Glycosylated hemoglobin is formed when linkages of glucose and related monosaccharides bind to hemoglobin A and its concentration represents the average blood glucose level over the previous several weeks. HbA1c levels are used as a measure of long-term control of plasma glucose (normal, 4 to 6 percent). In controlled diabetes mellitus, the concentration of glycosylated hemoglobin A is within the normal range, but in uncontrolled cases the level may be 3 to 4 times the normal conentration. Generally, complications are substantially lower among patients with Hb levels of 7 percent or less than in patients with HbA1c levels of 9 percent or more. [NIH]

Hemoglobinuria: The presence of free hemoglobin in the urine. [NIH]

Hemorrhage: Bleeding or escape of blood from a vessel. [NIH]

Hemostasis: The process which spontaneously arrests the flow of blood from vessels carrying blood under pressure. It is accomplished by contraction of the vessels, adhesion and aggregation of formed blood elements, and the process of blood or plasma coagulation. [NIH]

Hepatic: Refers to the liver. [NIH]

Hereditary: Of, relating to, or denoting factors that can be transmitted genetically from one generation to another. [NIH]

Heredity: 1. The genetic transmission of a particular quality or trait from parent to offspring. 2. The genetic constitution of an individual. [EU]

Heterogeneity: The property of one or more samples or populations which implies that they are not identical in respect of some or all of their parameters, e. g. heterogeneity of variance. [NIH]

Heterozygotes: Having unlike alleles at one or more corresponding loci on homologous chromosomes. [NIH]

Hirsutism: Excess hair in females and children with an adult male pattern of distribution. The concept does not include hypertrichosis, which is localized or generalized excess hair. [NIH]

Homeostasis: The processes whereby the internal environment of an organism tends to remain balanced and stable. [NIH]

Homologous: Corresponding in structure, position, origin, etc., as (a) the feathers of a bird and the scales of a fish, (b) antigen and its specific antibody, (c) allelic chromosomes. [EU]

Hormonal: Pertaining to or of the nature of a hormone. [EU]

Hormone: A substance in the body that regulates certain organs. Hormones such as gastrin help in breaking down food. Some hormones come from cells in the stomach and small intestine. [NIH]

Hormone Antagonists: Chemical substances which inhibit the function of the endocrine glands, the biosynthesis of their secreted hormones, or the action of hormones upon their specific sites. [NIH]

Hormone therapy: Treatment of cancer by removing, blocking, or adding hormones. Also called endocrine therapy. [NIH]

Horseradish Peroxidase: An enzyme isolated from horseradish which is able to act as an antigen. It is frequently used as a histochemical tracer for light and electron microscopy. Its antigenicity has permitted its use as a combined antigen and marker in experimental immunology. [NIH]

Hybrid: Cross fertilization between two varieties or, more usually, two species of vines, see also crossing. [NIH]

Hydrogen: The first chemical element in the periodic table. It has the atomic symbol H, atomic number 1, and atomic weight 1. It exists, under normal conditions, as a colorless, odorless, tasteless, diatomic gas. Hydrogen ions are protons. Besides the common H1 isotope, hydrogen exists as the stable isotope deuterium and the unstable, radioactive isotope tritium. [NIH]

Hydrophobic: Not readily absorbing water, or being adversely affected by water, as a hydrophobic colloid. [EU]

Hyperandrogenism: A state characterized or caused by an excessive secretion of androgens by the adrenal cortex, ovaries, or testes. The clinical significance in males is negligible, so the term is used most commonly with reference to the female. The common manifestations in women are hirsutism and virilism. It is often caused by ovarian disease (particularly the polycystic ovary syndrome) and by adrenal diseases (particularly adrenal gland hyperfunction). [NIH]

Hypercholesterolemia: Abnormally high levels of cholesterol in the blood. [NIH]

Hyperglycemia: Abnormally high blood sugar. [NIH]

Hyperlipidemia: An excess of lipids in the blood. [NIH]

Hyperplasia: An increase in the number of cells in a tissue or organ, not due to tumor formation. It differs from hypertrophy, which is an increase in bulk without an increase in the number of cells. [NIH]

Hypersecretion: Excessive secretion. [EU]

Hypersensitivity: Altered reactivity to an antigen, which can result in pathologic reactions upon subsequent exposure to that particular antigen. [NIH]

Hyperstimulation: Excessive stimulation. [EU]

Hypertension: Persistently high arterial blood pressure. Currently accepted threshold levels are 140 mm Hg systolic and 90 mm Hg diastolic pressure. [NIH]

Hyperthermia: A type of treatment in which body tissue is exposed to high temperatures to damage and kill cancer cells or to make cancer cells more sensitive to the effects of radiation and certain anticancer drugs. [NIH]

Hypertrichosis: Localized or generalized excess hair. The concept does not include hirsutism, which is excess hair in females and children with an adult male pattern of distribution. [NIH]

Hypertriglyceridemia: Condition of elevated triglyceride concentration in the blood; an inherited form occurs in familial hyperlipoproteinemia IIb and hyperlipoproteinemia type IV. It has been linked to higher risk of heart disease and arteriosclerosis. [NIH]

Hypertrophy: General increase in bulk of a part or organ, not due to tumor formation, nor to an increase in the number of cells. [NIH]

Hypogonadism: Condition resulting from or characterized by abnormally decreased functional activity of the gonads, with retardation of growth and sexual development. [NIH]

Hypothalamic: Of or involving the hypothalamus. [EU]

Hypothalamus: Ventral part of the diencephalon extending from the region of the optic chiasm to the caudal border of the mammillary bodies and forming the inferior and lateral walls of the third ventricle. [NIH]

Hypothyroidism: Deficiency of thyroid activity. In adults, it is most common in women and is characterized by decrease in basal metabolic rate, tiredness and lethargy, sensitivity to cold, and menstrual disturbances. If untreated, it progresses to full-blown myxoedema. In infants, severe hypothyroidism leads to cretinism. In juveniles, the manifestations are intermediate, with less severe mental and developmental retardation and only mild symptoms of the adult form. When due to pituitary deficiency of thyrotropin secretion it is called secondary hypothyroidism. [EU]

Id: The part of the personality structure which harbors the unconscious instinctive desires and strivings of the individual. [NIH]

Idiopathic: Describes a disease of unknown cause. [NIH]

Immune response: The activity of the immune system against foreign substances (antigens). [NIH]

Immunoassay: Immunochemical assay or detection of a substance by serologic or immunologic methods. Usually the substance being studied serves as antigen both in antibody production and in measurement of antibody by the test substance. [NIH]

Immunodeficiency: The decreased ability of the body to fight infection and disease. [NIH]

Immunology: The study of the body's immune system. [NIH]

Immunotherapy: Manipulation of the host's immune system in treatment of disease. It includes both active and passive immunization as well as immunosuppressive therapy to prevent graft rejection. [NIH]

Impairment: In the context of health experience, an impairment is any loss or abnormality of psychological, physiological, or anatomical structure or function. [NIH]

Implantation: The insertion or grafting into the body of biological, living, inert, or radioactive material. [EU]

In situ: In the natural or normal place; confined to the site of origin without invasion of neighbouring tissues. [EU]

In vitro: In the laboratory (outside the body). The opposite of in vivo (in the body). [NIH]

In vivo: In the body. The opposite of in vitro (outside the body or in the laboratory). [NIH]

Incision: A cut made in the body during surgery. [NIH]

Indicative: That indicates; that points out more or less exactly; that reveals fairly clearly. [EU]

Induction: The act or process of inducing or causing to occur, especially the production of a specific morphogenetic effect in the developing embryo through the influence of evocators or organizers, or the production of anaesthesia or unconsciousness by use of appropriate agents. [EU]

Infarction: A pathological process consisting of a sudden insufficient blood supply to an area, which results in necrosis of that area. It is usually caused by a thrombus, an embolus, or a vascular torsion. [NIH]

Infection: 1. Invasion and multiplication of microorganisms in body tissues, which may be clinically unapparent or result in local cellular injury due to competitive metabolism, toxins, intracellular replication, or antigen-antibody response. The infection may remain localized, subclinical, and temporary if the body's defensive mechanisms are effective. A local infection may persist and spread by extension to become an acute, subacute, or chronic clinical infection or disease state. A local infection may also become systemic when the microorganisms gain access to the lymphatic or vascular system. 2. An infectious disease. [EU]

Infertility: The diminished or absent ability to conceive or produce an offspring while sterility is the complete inability to conceive or produce an offspring. [NIH]

Inflammation: A pathological process characterized by injury or destruction of tissues caused by a variety of cytologic and chemical reactions. It is usually manifested by typical signs of pain, heat, redness, swelling, and loss of function. [NIH]

Infusion: A method of putting fluids, including drugs, into the bloodstream. Also called intravenous infusion. [NIH]

Ingestion: Taking into the body by mouth [NIH]

Inhibin: Glyceroprotein hormone produced in the seminiferous tubules by the Sertoli cells in the male and by the granulosa cells in the female follicles. The hormone inhibits FSH and LH synthesis and secretion by the pituitary cells thereby affecting sexual maturation and fertility. [NIH]

Initiation: Mutation induced by a chemical reactive substance causing cell changes; being a step in a carcinogenic process. [NIH]

Inositol: An isomer of glucose that has traditionally been considered to be a B vitamin although it has an uncertain status as a vitamin and a deficiency syndrome has not been identified in man. (From Martindale, The Extra Pharmacopoeia, 30th ed, p1379) Inositol phospholipids are important in signal transduction. [NIH]

Inotropic: Affecting the force or energy of muscular contractions. [EU]

Insight: The capacity to understand one's own motives, to be aware of one's own psychodynamics, to appreciate the meaning of symbolic behavior. [NIH]

Insomnia: Difficulty in going to sleep or getting enough sleep. [NIH]

Insulin: A protein hormone secreted by beta cells of the pancreas. Insulin plays a major role in the regulation of glucose metabolism, generally promoting the cellular utilization of glucose. It is also an important regulator of protein and lipid metabolism. Insulin is used as a drug to control insulin-dependent diabetes mellitus. [NIH]

Insulin-dependent diabetes mellitus: A disease characterized by high levels of blood glucose resulting from defects in insulin secretion, insulin action, or both. Autoimmune, genetic, and environmental factors are involved in the development of type I diabetes. [NIH]

Insulin-like: Muscular growth factor. [NIH]

Internal Medicine: A medical specialty concerned with the diagnosis and treatment of diseases of the internal organ systems of adults. [NIH]

Interstitial: Pertaining to or situated between parts or in the interspaces of a tissue. [EU]

Intestinal: Having to do with the intestines. [NIH]

Intestines: The section of the alimentary canal from the stomach to the anus. It includes the large intestine and small intestine. [NIH]

Intoxication: Poisoning, the state of being poisoned. [EU]

Intracellular: Inside a cell. [NIH]

Intravascular: Within a vessel or vessels. [EU]

Intravenous: IV. Into a vein. [NIH]

Intrinsic: Situated entirely within or pertaining exclusively to a part. [EU]

Invasive: 1. Having the quality of invasiveness. 2. Involving puncture or incision of the skin or insertion of an instrument or foreign material into the body; said of diagnostic techniques. [EU]

Involuntary: Reaction occurring without intention or volition. [NIH]

Ischemia: Deficiency of blood in a part, due to functional constriction or actual obstruction of a blood vessel. [EU]

Joint: The point of contact between elements of an animal skeleton with the parts that surround and support it. [NIH]

Kb: A measure of the length of DNA fragments, 1 Kb = 1000 base pairs. The largest DNA fragments are up to 50 kilobases long. [NIH]

Ketoconazole: Broad spectrum antifungal agent used for long periods at high doses, especially in immunosuppressed patients. [NIH]

Ketone Bodies: Chemicals that the body makes when there is not enough insulin in the blood and it must break down fat for its energy. Ketone bodies can poison and even kill body cells. When the body does not have the help of insulin, the ketones build up in the blood and then "spill" over into the urine so that the body can get rid of them. The body can also rid itself of one type of ketone, called acetone, through the lungs. This gives the breath a fruity odor. Ketones that build up in the body for a long time lead to serious illness and coma. [NIH]

Ketonuria: Having ketone bodies in the urine; a warning sign of diabetic ketoacidosis (DKA). [NIH]

Kidney Disease: Any one of several chronic conditions that are caused by damage to the cells of the kidney. People who have had diabetes for a long time may have kidney damage. Also called nephropathy. [NIH]

Lactation: The period of the secretion of milk. [EU]

Laparotomy: A surgical incision made in the wall of the abdomen. [NIH]

Large Intestine: The part of the intestine that goes from the cecum to the rectum. The large intestine absorbs water from stool and changes it from a liquid to a solid form. The large intestine is 5 feet long and includes the appendix, cecum, colon, and rectum. Also called colon. [NIH]

Leptin: A 16-kD peptide hormone secreted from white adipocytes and implicated in the regulation of food intake and energy balance. Leptin provides the key afferent signal from fat cells in the feedback system that controls body fat stores. [NIH]

Lethargy: Abnormal drowsiness or stupor; a condition of indifference. [EU]

Leucine: An essential branched-chain amino acid important for hemoglobin formation. [NIH]

Leucocyte: All the white cells of the blood and their precursors (myeloid cell series, lymphoid cell series) but commonly used to indicate granulocytes exclusive of lymphocytes. [NIH]

Leukaemia: An acute or chronic disease of unknown cause in man and other warm-blooded animals that involves the blood-forming organs, is characterized by an abnormal increase in the number of leucocytes in the tissues of the body with or without a corresponding increase of those in the circulating blood, and is classified according of the type leucocyte most prominently involved. [EU]

Leukemia: Cancer of blood-forming tissue. [NIH]

Leukotrienes: A family of biologically active compounds derived from arachidonic acid by oxidative metabolism through the 5-lipoxygenase pathway. They participate in host defense reactions and pathophysiological conditions such as immediate hypersensitivity and inflammation. They have potent actions on many essential organs and systems, including the cardiovascular, pulmonary, and central nervous system as well as the gastrointestinal tract and the immune system. [NIH]

Leuprolide: A potent and long acting analog of naturally occurring gonadotropin-releasing hormone (gonadorelin). Its action is similar to gonadorelin, which regulates the synthesis and release of pituitary gonadotropins. [NIH]

Levodopa: The naturally occurring form of dopa and the immediate precursor of dopamine. Unlike dopamine itself, it can be taken orally and crosses the blood-brain barrier. It is rapidly taken up by dopaminergic neurons and converted to dopamine. It is used for the treatment of parkinsonism and is usually given with agents that inhibit its conversion to dopamine outside of the central nervous system. [NIH]

Libido: The psychic drive or energy associated with sexual instinct in the broad sense (pleasure and love-object seeking). It may also connote the psychic energy associated with instincts in general that motivate behavior. [NIH]

Library Services: Services offered to the library user. They include reference and circulation. [NIH]

Ligament: A band of fibrous tissue that connects bones or cartilages, serving to support and strengthen joints. [EU]

Ligands: A RNA simulation method developed by the MIT. [NIH]

Linkage: The tendency of two or more genes in the same chromosome to remain together from one generation to the next more frequently than expected according to the law of independent assortment. [NIH]

Lipid: Fat. [NIH]

Lipoprotein: Any of the lipid-protein complexes in which lipids are transported in the blood; lipoprotein particles consist of a spherical hydrophobic core of triglycerides or cholesterol esters surrounded by an amphipathic monolayer of phospholipids, cholesterol, and apolipoproteins; the four principal classes are high-density, low-density, and very-low-density lipoproteins and chylomicrons. [EU]

Liposarcoma: A rare cancer of the fat cells. [NIH]

Liver: A large, glandular organ located in the upper abdomen. The liver cleanses the blood and aids in digestion by secreting bile. [NIH]

Liver Neoplasms: Tumors or cancer of the liver. [NIH]

Lobe: A portion of an organ such as the liver, lung, breast, or brain. [NIH]

Localization: The process of determining or marking the location or site of a lesion or disease. May also refer to the process of keeping a lesion or disease in a specific location or site. [NIH]

Localized: Cancer which has not metastasized yet. [NIH]

Low-density lipoprotein: Lipoprotein that contains most of the cholesterol in the blood. LDL carries cholesterol to the tissues of the body, including the arteries. A high level of LDL increases the risk of heart disease. LDL typically contains 60 to 70 percent of the total serum cholesterol and both are directly correlated with CHD risk. [NIH]

Luteal Phase: The period of the menstrual cycle that begins with ovulation and ends with menstruation. [NIH]

Lutein Cells: The cells of the corpus luteum which are derived from the granulosa cells and the theca cells of the Graafian follicle. [NIH]

Luteinizing hormone-releasing hormone agonist: LH-RH agonist. A drug that inhibits the secretion of sex hormones. In men, LH-RH agonist causes testosterone levels to fall. In women, LH-RH agonist causes the levels of estrogen and other sex hormones to fall. [NIH]

Lymph: The almost colorless fluid that travels through the lymphatic system and carries cells that help fight infection and disease. [NIH]

Lymph node: A rounded mass of lymphatic tissue that is surrounded by a capsule of connective tissue. Also known as a lymph gland. Lymph nodes are spread out along lymphatic vessels and contain many lymphocytes, which filter the lymphatic fluid (lymph). [NIH]

Lymphocyte: A white blood cell. Lymphocytes have a number of roles in the immune system, including the production of antibodies and other substances that fight infection and diseases. [NIH]

Lymphoid: Referring to lymphocytes, a type of white blood cell. Also refers to tissue in which lymphocytes develop. [NIH]

Lymphoma: A general term for various neoplastic diseases of the lymphoid tissue. [NIH]

Magnetic Resonance Imaging: Non-invasive method of demonstrating internal anatomy based on the principle that atomic nuclei in a strong magnetic field absorb pulses of radiofrequency energy and emit them as radiowaves which can be reconstructed into computerized images. The concept includes proton spin tomographic techniques. [NIH]

Major Histocompatibility Complex: The genetic region which contains the loci of genes which determine the structure of the serologically defined (SD) and lymphocyte-defined (LD) transplantation antigens, genes which control the structure of the immune response-associated (Ia) antigens, the immune response (Ir) genes which control the ability of an animal to respond immunologically to antigenic stimuli, and genes which determine the structure and/or level of the first four components of complement. [NIH]

Malabsorption: Impaired intestinal absorption of nutrients. [EU]

Malignancy: A cancerous tumor that can invade and destroy nearby tissue and spread to other parts of the body. [NIH]

Malignant: Cancerous; a growth with a tendency to invade and destroy nearby tissue and spread to other parts of the body. [NIH]

Malnutrition: A condition caused by not eating enough food or not eating a balanced diet. [NIH]

Manic: Affected with mania. [EU]

McMaster: Index used to measure painful syndromes linked to arthrosis. [NIH]

Medial: Lying near the midsaggital plane of the body; opposed to lateral. [NIH]

Mediate: Indirect; accomplished by the aid of an intervening medium. [EU]

Mediator: An object or substance by which something is mediated, such as (1) a structure of the nervous system that transmits impulses eliciting a specific response; (2) a chemical substance (transmitter substance) that induces activity in an excitable tissue, such as nerve or muscle; or (3) a substance released from cells as the result of the interaction of antigen with antibody or by the action of antigen with a sensitized lymphocyte. [EU]

Medical castration: Refers to the use of drugs to suppress the function of the ovaries or testicles. [NIH]

Medical Records: Recording of pertinent information concerning patient's illness or illnesses. [NIH]

MEDLINE: An online database of MEDLARS, the computerized bibliographic Medical Literature Analysis and Retrieval System of the National Library of Medicine. [NIH]

Meiosis: A special method of cell division, occurring in maturation of the germ cells, by means of which each daughter nucleus receives half the number of chromosomes characteristic of the somatic cells of the species. [NIH]

Melanocytes: Epidermal dendritic pigment cells which control long-term morphological color changes by alteration in their number or in the amount of pigment they produce and store in the pigment containing organelles called melanosomes. Melanophores are larger cells which do not exist in mammals. [NIH]

Melanoma: A form of skin cancer that arises in melanocytes, the cells that produce pigment. Melanoma usually begins in a mole. [NIH]

Melanosis: Disorders of increased melanin pigmentation that develop without preceding inflammatory disease. [NIH]

Membrane: A very thin layer of tissue that covers a surface. [NIH]

Menopause: Permanent cessation of menstruation. [NIH]

Menstrual Cycle: The period of the regularly recurring physiologic changes in the endometrium occurring during the reproductive period in human females and some primates and culminating in partial sloughing of the endometrium (menstruation). [NIH]

Menstruation: The normal physiologic discharge through the vagina of blood and mucosal tissues from the nonpregnant uterus. [NIH]

Mental: Pertaining to the mind; psychic. 2. (L. mentum chin) pertaining to the chin. [EU]

Mental Disorders: Psychiatric illness or diseases manifested by breakdowns in the adaptational process expressed primarily as abnormalities of thought, feeling, and behavior producing either distress or impairment of function. [NIH]

Mental Health: The state wherein the person is well adjusted. [NIH]

Mesoderm: The middle germ layer of the embryo. [NIH]

Meta-Analysis: A quantitative method of combining the results of independent studies (usually drawn from the published literature) and synthesizing summaries and conclusions which may be used to evaluate therapeutic effectiveness, plan new studies, etc., with application chiefly in the areas of research and medicine. [NIH]

Metabolic disorder: A condition in which normal metabolic processes are disrupted, usually because of a missing enzyme. [NIH]

Metaphase: The second phase of cell division, in which the chromosomes line up across the equatorial plane of the spindle prior to separation. [NIH]

Methionine: A sulfur containing essential amino acid that is important in many body functions. It is a chelating agent for heavy metals. [NIH]

Metoclopramide: A dopamine D2 antagonist that is used as an antiemetic. [NIH]

MI: Myocardial infarction. Gross necrosis of the myocardium as a result of interruption of the blood supply to the area; it is almost always caused by atherosclerosis of the coronary arteries, upon which coronary thrombosis is usually superimposed. [NIH]

Microorganism: An organism that can be seen only through a microscope. Microorganisms include bacteria, protozoa, algae, and fungi. Although viruses are not considered living organisms, they are sometimes classified as microorganisms. [NIH]

Migration: The systematic movement of genes between populations of the same species, geographic race, or variety. [NIH]

Mineralocorticoids: A group of corticosteroids primarily associated with the regulation of water and electrolyte balance. This is accomplished through the effect on ion transport in renal tubules, resulting in retention of sodium and loss of potassium. Mineralocorticoid secretion is itself regulated by plasma volume, serum potassium, and angiotensin II. [NIH]

Miscarriage: Spontaneous expulsion of the products of pregnancy before the middle of the second trimester. [NIH]

Mitosis: A method of indirect cell division by means of which the two daughter nuclei normally receive identical complements of the number of chromosomes of the somatic cells of the species. [NIH]

Mobility: Capability of movement, of being moved, or of flowing freely. [EU]

Modeling: A treatment procedure whereby the therapist presents the target behavior which the learner is to imitate and make part of his repertoire. [NIH]

Modification: A change in an organism, or in a process in an organism, that is acquired from its own activity or environment. [NIH]

Molecular: Of, pertaining to, or composed of molecules : a very small mass of matter. [EU]

Molecule: A chemical made up of two or more atoms. The atoms in a molecule can be the same (an oxygen molecule has two oxygen atoms) or different (a water molecule has two hydrogen atoms and one oxygen atom). Biological molecules, such as proteins and DNA, can be made up of many thousands of atoms. [NIH]

Monitor: An apparatus which automatically records such physiological signs as respiration, pulse, and blood pressure in an anesthetized patient or one undergoing surgical or other procedures. [NIH]

Monocyte: A type of white blood cell. [NIH]

Monotherapy: A therapy which uses only one drug. [EU]

Morphological: Relating to the configuration or the structure of live organs. [NIH]

Morphology: The science of the form and structure of organisms (plants, animals, and other forms of life). [NIH]

Morula: The early embryo at the developmental stage in which the blastomeres, resulting from repeated mitotic divisions of the fertilized ovum, form a compact mass. [NIH]

Mucolytic: Destroying or dissolving mucin; an agent that so acts : a mucopolysaccharide or glycoprotein, the chief constituent of mucus. [EU]

Mucosa: A mucous membrane, or tunica mucosa. [EU]

Mucus: The viscous secretion of mucous membranes. It contains mucin, white blood cells, water, inorganic salts, and exfoliated cells. [NIH]

Muscle Fibers: Large single cells, either cylindrical or prismatic in shape, that form the basic unit of muscle tissue. They consist of a soft contractile substance enclosed in a tubular sheath. [NIH]

Muscular Atrophy: Derangement in size and number of muscle fibers occurring with aging, reduction in blood supply, or following immobilization, prolonged weightlessness, malnutrition, and particularly in denervation. [NIH]

Muscular Dystrophies: A general term for a group of inherited disorders which are characterized by progressive degeneration of skeletal muscles. [NIH]

Myocardium: The muscle tissue of the heart composed of striated, involuntary muscle known as cardiac muscle. [NIH]

Myotonic Dystrophy: A condition presenting muscle weakness and wasting which may be progressive. [NIH]

Naloxone: A specific opiate antagonist that has no agonist activity. It is a competitive antagonist at mu, delta, and kappa opioid receptors. [NIH]

Naltrexone: Derivative of noroxymorphone that is the N-cyclopropylmethyl congener of naloxone. It is a narcotic antagonist that is effective orally, longer lasting and more potent than naloxone, and has been proposed for the treatment of heroin addiction. The FDA has approved naltrexone for the treatment of alcohol dependence. [NIH]

Narcotic: 1. Pertaining to or producing narcosis. 2. An agent that produces insensibility or stupor, applied especially to the opioids, i.e. to any natural or synthetic drug that has morphine-like actions. [EU]

Nausea: An unpleasant sensation in the stomach usually accompanied by the urge to vomit. Common causes are early pregnancy, sea and motion sickness, emotional stress, intense pain, food poisoning, and various enteroviruses. [NIH]

NCI: National Cancer Institute. NCI, part of the National Institutes of Health of the United States Department of Health and Human Services, is the federal government's principal agency for cancer research. NCI conducts, coordinates, and funds cancer research, training, health information dissemination, and other programs with respect to the cause, diagnosis, prevention, and treatment of cancer. Access the NCI Web site at http://cancer.gov. [NIH]

Need: A state of tension or dissatisfaction felt by an individual that impels him to action toward a goal he believes will satisfy the impulse. [NIH]

Neonatal: Pertaining to the first four weeks after birth. [EU]

Neoplasia: Abnormal and uncontrolled cell growth. [NIH]

Neoplastic: Pertaining to or like a neoplasm (= any new and abnormal growth); pertaining to neoplasia (= the formation of a neoplasm). [EU]

Nephropathy: Disease of the kidneys. [EU]

Nerve: A cordlike structure of nervous tissue that connects parts of the nervous system with other tissues of the body and conveys nervous impulses to, or away from, these tissues. [NIH]

Nerve Growth Factor: Nerve growth factor is the first of a series of neurotrophic factors that were found to influence the growth and differentiation of sympathetic and sensory neurons. It is comprised of alpha, beta, and gamma subunits. The beta subunit is responsible for its growth stimulating activity. [NIH]

Nervous System: The entire nerve apparatus composed of the brain, spinal cord, nerves and ganglia. [NIH]

Neural: 1. Pertaining to a nerve or to the nerves. 2. Situated in the region of the spinal axis, as the neutral arch. [EU]

Neural Pathways: Neural tracts connecting one part of the nervous system with another. [NIH]

Neuroendocrine: Having to do with the interactions between the nervous system and the endocrine system. Describes certain cells that release hormones into the blood in response to stimulation of the nervous system. [NIH]

Neuronal: Pertaining to a neuron or neurons (= conducting cells of the nervous system). [EU]

Neurons: The basic cellular units of nervous tissue. Each neuron consists of a body, an axon, and dendrites. Their purpose is to receive, conduct, and transmit impulses in the nervous system. [NIH]

Neuropeptide: A member of a class of protein-like molecules made in the brain. Neuropeptides consist of short chains of amino acids, with some functioning as neurotransmitters and some functioning as hormones. [NIH]

Neurosecretory Systems: A system of neurons that has the specialized function to produce and secrete hormones, and that constitutes, in whole or in part, an endocrine organ or system. [NIH]

Neurotransmitter: Any of a group of substances that are released on excitation from the axon terminal of a presynaptic neuron of the central or peripheral nervous system and travel across the synaptic cleft to either excite or inhibit the target cell. Among the many substances that have the properties of a neurotransmitter are acetylcholine, norepinephrine, epinephrine, dopamine, glycine, y-aminobutyrate, glutamic acid, substance P, enkephalins, endorphins, and serotonin. [EU]

Nidation: Implantation of the conceptus in the endometrium. [EU]

Nitrogen: An element with the atomic symbol N, atomic number 7, and atomic weight 14. Nitrogen exists as a diatomic gas and makes up about 78% of the earth's atmosphere by volume. It is a constituent of proteins and nucleic acids and found in all living cells. [NIH]

Norepinephrine: Precursor of epinephrine that is secreted by the adrenal medulla and is a widespread central and autonomic neurotransmitter. Norepinephrine is the principal transmitter of most postganglionic sympathetic fibers and of the diffuse projection system in the brain arising from the locus ceruleus. It is also found in plants and is used pharmacologically as a sympathomimetic. [NIH]

Nuclear: A test of the structure, blood flow, and function of the kidneys. The doctor injects a mildly radioactive solution into an arm vein and uses x-rays to monitor its progress through the kidneys. [NIH]

Nuclei: A body of specialized protoplasm found in nearly all cells and containing the chromosomes. [NIH]

Nucleic acid: Either of two types of macromolecule (DNA or RNA) formed by polymerization of nucleotides. Nucleic acids are found in all living cells and contain the information (genetic code) for the transfer of genetic information from one generation to the next. [NIH]

Nucleus: A body of specialized protoplasm found in nearly all cells and containing the chromosomes. [NIH]

Nurse Practitioners: Nurses who are specially trained to assume an expanded role in providing medical care under the supervision of a physician. [NIH]

Occupational Health: The promotion and maintenance of physical and mental health in the work environment. [NIH]

Occupational Health Nursing: The practice of nursing in the work environment. [NIH]

Oestradiol: Growth hormone. [NIH]

Oligo: Chemical and mineral elements that exist in minimal (oligo) quantities in the body, in foods, in the air, in soil; name applied to any element observed as a microconstituent of plant or animal tissue and of beneficial, harmful, or even doubtful significance. [NIH]

Oligomenorrhea: Abnormally infrequent menstruation. [NIH]

Oncogene: A gene that normally directs cell growth. If altered, an oncogene can promote or allow the uncontrolled growth of cancer. Alterations can be inherited or caused by an environmental exposure to carcinogens. [NIH]

Only Child: Child who has no siblings. [NIH]

Oocytes: Female germ cells in stages between the prophase of the first maturation division and the completion of the second maturation division. [NIH]

Opacity: Degree of density (area most dense taken for reading). [NIH]

Ophthalmic: Pertaining to the eye. [EU]

Opiate: A remedy containing or derived from opium; also any drug that induces sleep. [EU]

Opium: The air-dried exudate from the unripe seed capsule of the opium poppy, Papaver somniferum, or its variant, P. album. It contains a number of alkaloids, but only a few - morphine, codeine, and papaverine - have clinical significance. Opium has been used as an analgesic, antitussive, antidiarrheal, and antispasmodic. [NIH]

Opsin: A protein formed, together with retinene, by the chemical breakdown of meta-rhodopsin. [NIH]

Optic Chiasm: The X-shaped structure formed by the meeting of the two optic nerves. At the optic chiasm the fibers from the medial part of each retina cross to project to the other side of the brain while the lateral retinal fibers continue on the same side. As a result each half of the brain receives information about the contralateral visual field from both eyes. [NIH]

Optic Nerve: The 2nd cranial nerve. The optic nerve conveys visual information from the retina to the brain. The nerve carries the axons of the retinal ganglion cells which sort at the optic chiasm and continue via the optic tracts to the brain. The largest projection is to the lateral geniculate nuclei; other important targets include the superior colliculi and the suprachiasmatic nuclei. Though known as the second cranial nerve, it is considered part of the central nervous system. [NIH]

Organelles: Specific particles of membrane-bound organized living substances present in eukaryotic cells, such as the mitochondria; the golgi apparatus; endoplasmic reticulum; lysomomes; plastids; and vacuoles. [NIH]

Ovarian Cysts: General term for cysts and cystic diseases of the ovary. [NIH]

Ovarian Follicle: Spheroidal cell aggregation in the ovary containing an ovum. It consists of an external fibro-vascular coat, an internal coat of nucleated cells, and a transparent, albuminous fluid in which the ovum is suspended. [NIH]

Ovarian Hyperstimulation Syndrome: Syndrome composed of a combination of ovarian enlargement and an acute fluid shift out of the intravascular space. The enlargement is caused by ovarian cyst formation and the fluid shift may result in ascites, hydrothorax, or generalized edema. The syndrome is most usually seen as a complication of ovulation induction, a treatment for infertility. [NIH]

Ovaries: The pair of female reproductive glands in which the ova, or eggs, are formed. The ovaries are located in the pelvis, one on each side of the uterus. [NIH]

Ovary: Either of the paired glands in the female that produce the female germ cells and secrete some of the female sex hormones. [NIH]

Overweight: An excess of body weight but not necessarily body fat; a body mass index of 25 to 29.9 kg/m2. [NIH]

Ovulation: The discharge of a secondary oocyte from a ruptured graafian follicle. [NIH]

Ovulation Induction: Techniques for the artifical induction of ovulation. [NIH]

Ovum: A female germ cell extruded from the ovary at ovulation. [NIH]

Ovum Implantation: Endometrial implantation of the blastocyst. [NIH]

Oxidation: The act of oxidizing or state of being oxidized. Chemically it consists in the increase of positive charges on an atom or the loss of negative charges. Most biological oxidations are accomplished by the removal of a pair of hydrogen atoms (dehydrogenation) from a molecule. Such oxidations must be accompanied by reduction of an acceptor molecule. Univalent o. indicates loss of one electron; divalent o., the loss of two electrons. [EU]

Palliative: 1. Affording relief, but not cure. 2. An alleviating medicine. [EU]

Pancreas: A mixed exocrine and endocrine gland situated transversely across the posterior abdominal wall in the epigastric and hypochondriac regions. The endocrine portion is comprised of the Islets of Langerhans, while the exocrine portion is a compound acinar gland that secretes digestive enzymes. [NIH]

Pancreatic: Having to do with the pancreas. [NIH]

Pancreatic cancer: Cancer of the pancreas, a salivary gland of the abdomen. [NIH]

Paroxysmal: Recurring in paroxysms (= spasms or seizures). [EU]

Parturition: The act or process of given birth to a child. [EU]

Pathogenesis: The cellular events and reactions that occur in the development of disease. [NIH]

Pathologic: 1. Indicative of or caused by a morbid condition. 2. Pertaining to pathology (= branch of medicine that treats the essential nature of the disease, especially the structural and functional changes in tissues and organs of the body caused by the disease). [EU]

Pathologic Processes: The abnormal mechanisms and forms involved in the dysfunctions of tissues and organs. [NIH]

Pathophysiology: Altered functions in an individual or an organ due to disease. [NIH]

Pelvic: Pertaining to the pelvis. [EU]

Pelvis: The lower part of the abdomen, located between the hip bones. [NIH]

Penis: The external reproductive organ of males. It is composed of a mass of erectile tissue enclosed in three cylindrical fibrous compartments. Two of the three compartments, the corpus cavernosa, are placed side-by-side along the upper part of the organ. The third compartment below, the corpus spongiosum, houses the urethra. [NIH]

Peptide: Any compound consisting of two or more amino acids, the building blocks of proteins. Peptides are combined to make proteins. [NIH]

Peripheral Nervous System: The nervous system outside of the brain and spinal cord. The peripheral nervous system has autonomic and somatic divisions. The autonomic nervous system includes the enteric, parasympathetic, and sympathetic subdivisions. The somatic nervous system includes the cranial and spinal nerves and their ganglia and the peripheral sensory receptors. [NIH]

Peristalsis: The rippling motion of muscles in the intestine or other tubular organs characterized by the alternate contraction and relaxation of the muscles that propel the contents onward. [NIH]

Pharmacologic: Pertaining to pharmacology or to the properties and reactions of drugs. [EU]

Phenotype: The outward appearance of the individual. It is the product of interactions between genes and between the genotype and the environment. This includes the killer phenotype, characteristic of yeasts. [NIH]

Phenyl: Ingredient used in cold and flu remedies. [NIH]

Phenytoin: An anticonvulsant that is used in a wide variety of seizures. It is also an anti-arrhythmic and a muscle relaxant. The mechanism of therapeutic action is not clear, although several cellular actions have been described including effects on ion channels, active transport, and general membrane stabilization. The mechanism of its muscle relaxant effect appears to involve a reduction in the sensitivity of muscle spindles to stretch. Phenytoin has been proposed for several other therapeutic uses, but its use has been limited by its many adverse effects and interactions with other drugs. [NIH]

Phospholipases: A class of enzymes that catalyze the hydrolysis of phosphoglycerides or glycerophosphatidates. EC 3.1.-. [NIH]

Phospholipids: Lipids containing one or more phosphate groups, particularly those derived from either glycerol (phosphoglycerides; glycerophospholipids) or sphingosine (sphingolipids). They are polar lipids that are of great importance for the structure and function of cell membranes and are the most abundant of membrane lipids, although not stored in large amounts in the system. [NIH]

Phosphorus: A non-metallic element that is found in the blood, muscles, nevers, bones, and teeth, and is a component of adenosine triphosphate (ATP; the primary energy source for the body's cells.) [NIH]

Phosphorylated: Attached to a phosphate group. [NIH]

Phosphorylation: The introduction of a phosphoryl group into a compound through the formation of an ester bond between the compound and a phosphorus moiety. [NIH]

Physical Examination: Systematic and thorough inspection of the patient for physical signs of disease or abnormality. [NIH]

Physiologic: Having to do with the functions of the body. When used in the phrase "physiologic age," it refers to an age assigned by general health, as opposed to calendar age. [NIH]

Physiology: The science that deals with the life processes and functions of organismus, their cells, tissues, and organs. [NIH]

Pigments: Any normal or abnormal coloring matter in plants, animals, or micro-organisms. [NIH]

Pilot study: The initial study examining a new method or treatment. [NIH]

Pituitary Gland: A small, unpaired gland situated in the sella turcica tissue. It is connected to the hypothalamus by a short stalk. [NIH]

Placenta: A highly vascular fetal organ through which the fetus absorbs oxygen and other nutrients and excretes carbon dioxide and other wastes. It begins to form about the eighth day of gestation when the blastocyst adheres to the decidua. [NIH]

Plants: Multicellular, eukaryotic life forms of the kingdom Plantae. They are characterized by a mainly photosynthetic mode of nutrition; essentially unlimited growth at localized regions of cell divisions (meristems); cellulose within cells providing rigidity; the absence of organs of locomotion; absense of nervous and sensory systems; and an alteration of haploid and diploid generations. [NIH]

Plaque: A clear zone in a bacterial culture grown on an agar plate caused by localized destruction of bacterial cells by a bacteriophage. The concentration of infective virus in a fluid can be estimated by applying the fluid to a culture and counting the number of. [NIH]

Plasma: The clear, yellowish, fluid part of the blood that carries the blood cells. The proteins that form blood clots are in plasma. [NIH]

Plasma protein: One of the hundreds of different proteins present in blood plasma, including carrier proteins (such albumin, transferrin, and haptoglobin), fibrinogen and other coagulation factors, complement components, immunoglobulins, enzyme inhibitors, precursors of substances such as angiotension and bradykinin, and many other types of proteins. [EU]

Plasmin: A product of the lysis of plasminogen (profibrinolysin) by plasminogen activators. It is composed of two polypeptide chains, light (B) and heavy (A), with a molecular weight of 75,000. It is the major proteolytic enzyme involved in blood clot retraction or the lysis of fibrin and quickly inactivated by antiplasmins. EC 3.4.21.7. [NIH]

Plasminogen: Precursor of fibrinolysin (plasmin). It is a single-chain beta-globulin of molecular weight 80-90,000 found mostly in association with fibrinogen in plasma; plasminogen activators change it to fibrinolysin. It is used in wound debriding and has been investigated as a thrombolytic agent. [NIH]

Platelet Activation: A series of progressive, overlapping events triggered by exposure of the platelets to subendothelial tissue. These events include shape change, adhesiveness, aggregation, and release reactions. When carried through to completion, these events lead to the formation of a stable hemostatic plug. [NIH]

Pneumonia: Inflammation of the lungs. [NIH]

Polycystic: An inherited disorder characterized by many grape-like clusters of fluid-filled cysts that make both kidneys larger over time. These cysts take over and destroy working kidney tissue. PKD may cause chronic renal failure and end-stage renal disease. [NIH]

Polycystic Ovary Syndrome: Clinical symptom complex characterized by oligomenorrhea or amenorrhea, anovulation, and regularly associated with bilateral polycystic ovaries. [NIH]

Polydipsia: Chronic excessive thirst, as in diabetes mellitus or diabetes insipidus. [EU]

Polymorphism: The occurrence together of two or more distinct forms in the same population. [NIH]

Polyphagia: Great hunger; a sign of diabetes. People with this great hunger often lose weight. [NIH]

Polysaccharide: A type of carbohydrate. It contains sugar molecules that are linked together chemically. [NIH]

Polyuria: Urination of a large volume of urine with an increase in urinary frequency, commonly seen in diabetes. [NIH]

Posterior: Situated in back of, or in the back part of, or affecting the back or dorsal surface of the body. In lower animals, it refers to the caudal end of the body. [EU]

Postnatal: Occurring after birth, with reference to the newborn. [EU]

Postprandial: Occurring after dinner, or after a meal; postcibal. [EU]

Postsynaptic: Nerve potential generated by an inhibitory hyperpolarizing stimulation. [NIH]

Post-translational: The cleavage of signal sequence that directs the passage of the protein through a cell or organelle membrane. [NIH]

Potassium: An element that is in the alkali group of metals. It has an atomic symbol K, atomic number 19, and atomic weight 39.10. It is the chief cation in the intracellular fluid of muscle and other cells. Potassium ion is a strong electrolyte and it plays a significant role in the regulation of fluid volume and maintenance of the water-electrolyte balance. [NIH]

Potentiation: An overall effect of two drugs taken together which is greater than the sum of the effects of each drug taken alone. [NIH]

Practicability: A non-standard characteristic of an analytical procedure. It is dependent on the scope of the method and is determined by requirements such as sample throughout and costs. [NIH]

Practice Guidelines: Directions or principles presenting current or future rules of policy for the health care practitioner to assist him in patient care decisions regarding diagnosis, therapy, or related clinical circumstances. The guidelines may be developed by government agencies at any level, institutions, professional societies, governing boards, or by the convening of expert panels. The guidelines form a basis for the evaluation of all aspects of health care and delivery. [NIH]

Preclinical: Before a disease becomes clinically recognizable. [EU]

Precursor: Something that precedes. In biological processes, a substance from which another, usually more active or mature substance is formed. In clinical medicine, a sign or symptom that heralds another. [EU]

Preeclampsia: A toxaemia of late pregnancy characterized by hypertension, edema, and proteinuria, when convulsions and coma are associated, it is called eclampsia. [EU]

Pregnancy Complications: The co-occurrence of pregnancy and a disease. The disease may precede or follow conception and it may or may not have a deleterious effect on the pregnant woman or fetus. [NIH]

Pregnancy Outcome: Results of conception and ensuing pregnancy, including live birth, stillbirth, spontaneous abortion, induced abortion. The outcome may follow natural or artificial insemination or any of the various reproduction techniques, such as embryo transfer or fertilization in vitro. [NIH]

Premenstrual: Occurring before menstruation. [EU]

Premenstrual Syndrome: A syndrome occurring most often during the last week of the menstrual cycle and ending soon after the onset of menses. Some of the symptoms are emotional instability, insomnia, headache, nausea, vomiting, abdominal distension, and painful breasts. [NIH]

Prenatal: Existing or occurring before birth, with reference to the fetus. [EU]

Preoptic Area: Region of hypothalamus between the anterior commissure and optic chiasm. [NIH]

Presynaptic: Situated proximal to a synapse, or occurring before the synapse is crossed. [EU]

Prevalence: The total number of cases of a given disease in a specified population at a designated time. It is differentiated from incidence, which refers to the number of new cases in the population at a given time. [NIH]

Progesterone: Pregn-4-ene-3,20-dione. The principal progestational hormone of the body, secreted by the corpus luteum, adrenal cortex, and placenta. Its chief function is to prepare the uterus for the reception and development of the fertilized ovum. It acts as an antiovulatory agent when administered on days 5-25 of the menstrual cycle. [NIH]

Progestogen: A term applied to any substance possessing progestational activity. [EU]

Progression: Increase in the size of a tumor or spread of cancer in the body. [NIH]

Progressive: Advancing; going forward; going from bad to worse; increasing in scope or severity. [EU]

Prolactin: Pituitary lactogenic hormone. A polypeptide hormone with a molecular weight of about 23,000. It is essential in the induction of lactation in mammals at parturition and is synergistic with estrogen. The hormone also brings about the release of progesterone from lutein cells, which renders the uterine mucosa suited for the embedding of the ovum should fertilization occur. [NIH]

Promoter: A chemical substance that increases the activity of a carcinogenic process. [NIH]

Prophase: The first phase of cell division, in which the chromosomes become visible, the nucleus starts to lose its identity, the spindle appears, and the centrioles migrate toward opposite poles. [NIH]

Proportional: Being in proportion : corresponding in size, degree, or intensity, having the same or a constant ratio; of, relating to, or used in determining proportions. [EU]

Prospective study: An epidemiologic study in which a group of individuals (a cohort), all free of a particular disease and varying in their exposure to a possible risk factor, is followed over a specific amount of time to determine the incidence rates of the disease in the exposed and unexposed groups. [NIH]

Prostaglandin: Any of a group of components derived from unsaturated 20-carbon fatty acids, primarily arachidonic acid, via the cyclooxygenase pathway that are extremely potent mediators of a diverse group of physiologic processes. The abbreviation for prostaglandin is PG; specific compounds are designated by adding one of the letters A through I to indicate the type of substituents found on the hydrocarbon skeleton and a subscript (1, 2 or 3) to indicate the number of double bonds in the hydrocarbon skeleton e.g., PGE2. The predominant naturally occurring prostaglandins all have two double bonds and are synthesized from arachidonic acid (5,8,11,14-eicosatetraenoic acid) by the pathway shown in the illustration. The 1 series and 3 series are produced by the same pathway with fatty acids having one fewer double bond (8,11,14-eicosatrienoic acid or one more double bond (5,8,11,14,17-eicosapentaenoic acid) than arachidonic acid. The subscript a or ß indicates the configuration at C-9 (a denotes a substituent below the plane of the ring, ß, above the plane). The naturally occurring PGF's have the a configuration, e.g., PGF2a. All of the prostaglandins act by binding to specific cell-surface receptors causing an increase in the level of the intracellular second messenger cyclic AMP (and in some cases cyclic GMP also). The effect produced by the cyclic AMP increase depends on the specific cell type. In some cases there is also a positive feedback effect. Increased cyclic AMP increases prostaglandin synthesis leading to further increases in cyclic AMP. [EU]

Prostaglandins A: (13E,15S)-15-Hydroxy-9-oxoprosta-10,13-dien-1-oic acid (PGA(1)); (5Z,13E,15S)-15-hydroxy-9-oxoprosta-5,10,13-trien-1-oic acid (PGA(2)); (5Z,13E,15S,17Z)-15-hydroxy-9-oxoprosta-5,10,13,17-tetraen-1-oic acid (PGA(3)). A group of naturally occurring secondary prostaglandins derived from PGE. PGA(1) and PGA(2) as well as their 19-hydroxy derivatives are found in many organs and tissues. [NIH]

Prostate: A gland in males that surrounds the neck of the bladder and the urethra. It secretes a substance that liquifies coagulated semen. It is situated in the pelvic cavity behind the lower part of the pubic symphysis, above the deep layer of the triangular ligament, and rests upon the rectum. [NIH]

Protease: Proteinase (= any enzyme that catalyses the splitting of interior peptide bonds in a protein). [EU]

Protective Agents: Synthetic or natural substances which are given to prevent a disease or disorder or are used in the process of treating a disease or injury due to a poisonous agent. [NIH]

Protein C: A vitamin-K dependent zymogen present in the blood, which, upon activation by thrombin and thrombomodulin exerts anticoagulant properties by inactivating factors Va and VIIIa at the rate-limiting steps of thrombin formation. [NIH]

Protein S: The vitamin K-dependent cofactor of activated protein C. Together with protein C, it inhibits the action of factors VIIIa and Va. A deficiency in protein S can lead to recurrent venous and arterial thrombosis. [NIH]

Proteins: Polymers of amino acids linked by peptide bonds. The specific sequence of amino acids determines the shape and function of the protein. [NIH]

Proteinuria: The presence of protein in the urine, indicating that the kidneys are not working properly. [NIH]

Proteolytic: 1. Pertaining to, characterized by, or promoting proteolysis. 2. An enzyme that promotes proteolysis (= the splitting of proteins by hydrolysis of the peptide bonds with formation of smaller polypeptides). [EU]

Psychic: Pertaining to the psyche or to the mind; mental. [EU]

Psychomotor: Pertaining to motor effects of cerebral or psychic activity. [EU]

Puberty: The period during which the secondary sex characteristics begin to develop and the capability of sexual reproduction is attained. [EU]

Public Health: Branch of medicine concerned with the prevention and control of disease and disability, and the promotion of physical and mental health of the population on the international, national, state, or municipal level. [NIH]

Public Policy: A course or method of action selected, usually by a government, from among alternatives to guide and determine present and future decisions. [NIH]

Pulmonary: Relating to the lungs. [NIH]

Pulmonary Artery: The short wide vessel arising from the conus arteriosus of the right ventricle and conveying unaerated blood to the lungs. [NIH]

Pulmonary hypertension: Abnormally high blood pressure in the arteries of the lungs. [NIH]

Pulse: The rhythmical expansion and contraction of an artery produced by waves of pressure caused by the ejection of blood from the left ventricle of the heart as it contracts. [NIH]

Quality of Life: A generic concept reflecting concern with the modification and enhancement of life attributes, e.g., physical, political, moral and social environment. [NIH]

Race: A population within a species which exhibits general similarities within itself, but is both discontinuous and distinct from other populations of that species, though not sufficiently so as to achieve the status of a taxon. [NIH]

Racemic: Optically inactive but resolvable in the way of all racemic compounds. [NIH]

Radiation: Emission or propagation of electromagnetic energy (waves/rays), or the waves/rays themselves; a stream of electromagnetic particles (electrons, neutrons, protons, alpha particles) or a mixture of these. The most common source is the sun. [NIH]

Radio Waves: That portion of the electromagnetic spectrum beyond the microwaves, with wavelengths as high as 30 KM. They are used in communications, including television. Short Wave or HF (high frequency), UHF (ultrahigh frequency) and VHF (very high frequency) waves are used in citizen's band communication. [NIH]

Radioactive: Giving off radiation. [NIH]

Radiopharmaceutical: Any medicinal product which, when ready for use, contains one or more radionuclides (radioactive isotopes) included for a medicinal purpose. [NIH]

Randomized: Describes an experiment or clinical trial in which animal or human subjects are assigned by chance to separate groups that compare different treatments. [NIH]

Receptivity: The condition of the reproductive organs of a female flower that permits effective pollination. [NIH]

Receptor: A molecule inside or on the surface of a cell that binds to a specific substance and causes a specific physiologic effect in the cell. [NIH]

Receptors, Steroid: Proteins found usually in the cytoplasm or nucleus that specifically bind steroid hormones and trigger changes influencing the behavior of cells. The steroid receptor-steroid hormone complex regulates the transcription of specific genes. [NIH]

Recombinant: A cell or an individual with a new combination of genes not found together in either parent; usually applied to linked genes. [EU]

Rectum: The last 8 to 10 inches of the large intestine. [NIH]

Recurrence: The return of a sign, symptom, or disease after a remission. [NIH]

Red Nucleus: A pinkish-yellow portion of the midbrain situated in the rostral mesencephalic tegmentum. It receives a large projection from the contralateral half of the cerebellum via the superior cerebellar peduncle and a projection from the ipsilateral motor cortex. [NIH]

Reductase: Enzyme converting testosterone to dihydrotestosterone. [NIH]

Refer: To send or direct for treatment, aid, information, de decision. [NIH]

Refraction: A test to determine the best eyeglasses or contact lenses to correct a refractive error (myopia, hyperopia, or astigmatism). [NIH]

Regimen: A treatment plan that specifies the dosage, the schedule, and the duration of treatment. [NIH]

Remission: A decrease in or disappearance of signs and symptoms of cancer. In partial remission, some, but not all, signs and symptoms of cancer have disappeared. In complete remission, all signs and symptoms of cancer have disappeared, although there still may be cancer in the body. [NIH]

Renin: An enzyme which is secreted by the kidney and is formed from prorenin in plasma and kidney. The enzyme cleaves the Leu-Leu bond in angiotensinogen to generate angiotensin I. EC 3.4.23.15. (Formerly EC 3.4.99.19). [NIH]

Renin-Angiotensin System: A system consisting of renin, angiotensin-converting enzyme, and angiotensin II. Renin, an enzyme produced in the kidney, acts on angiotensinogen, an alpha-2 globulin produced by the liver, forming angiotensin I. The converting enzyme contained in the lung acts on angiotensin I in the plasma converting it to angiotensin II, the most powerful directly pressor substance known. It causes contraction of the arteriolar smooth muscle and has other indirect actions mediated through the adrenal cortex. [NIH]

Reproduction Techniques: Methods pertaining to the generation of new individuals. [NIH]

Reproductive cells: Egg and sperm cells. Each mature reproductive cell carries a single set of 23 chromosomes. [NIH]

Reproductive system: In women, this system includes the ovaries, the fallopian tubes, the uterus (womb), the cervix, and the vagina (birth canal). The reproductive system in men includes the prostate, the testes, and the penis. [NIH]

Resection: Removal of tissue or part or all of an organ by surgery. [NIH]

Respiration: The act of breathing with the lungs, consisting of inspiration, or the taking into the lungs of the ambient air, and of expiration, or the expelling of the modified air which contains more carbon dioxide than the air taken in (Blakiston's Gould Medical Dictionary, 4th ed.). This does not include tissue respiration (= oxygen consumption) or cell respiration (= cell respiration). [NIH]

Retina: The ten-layered nervous tissue membrane of the eye. It is continuous with the optic nerve and receives images of external objects and transmits visual impulses to the brain. Its outer surface is in contact with the choroid and the inner surface with the vitreous body. The outer-most layer is pigmented, whereas the inner nine layers are transparent. [NIH]

Retinal: 1. Pertaining to the retina. 2. The aldehyde of retinol, derived by the oxidative enzymatic splitting of absorbed dietary carotene, and having vitamin A activity. In the retina, retinal combines with opsins to form visual pigments. One isomer, 11-cis retinal combines with opsin in the rods (scotopsin) to form rhodopsin, or visual purple. Another, all-trans retinal (trans-r.); visual yellow; xanthopsin) results from the bleaching of rhodopsin by light, in which the 11-cis form is converted to the all-trans form. Retinal also combines with opsins in the cones (photopsins) to form the three pigments responsible for colour vision. Called also retinal, and retinene1. [EU]

Retinal Vein: Central retinal vein and its tributaries. It runs a short course within the optic nerve and then leaves and empties into the superior ophthalmic vein or cavernous sinus. [NIH]

Retinal Vein Occlusion: Occlusion of the retinal vein. Those at high risk for this condition include patients with hypertension, diabetes mellitus, arteriosclerosis, and other cardiovascular diseases. [NIH]

Retinoblastoma: An eye cancer that most often occurs in children younger than 5 years. It occurs in hereditary and nonhereditary (sporadic) forms. [NIH]

Retinol: Vitamin A. It is essential for proper vision and healthy skin and mucous membranes. Retinol is being studied for cancer prevention; it belongs to the family of drugs called retinoids. [NIH]

Retroperitoneal: Having to do with the area outside or behind the peritoneum (the tissue that lines the abdominal wall and covers most of the organs in the abdomen). [NIH]

Retrospective: Looking back at events that have already taken place. [NIH]

Retrospective study: A study that looks backward in time, usually using medical records and interviews with patients who already have or had a disease. [NIH]

Rhodopsin: A photoreceptor protein found in retinal rods. It is a complex formed by the binding of retinal, the oxidized form of retinol, to the protein opsin and undergoes a series of complex reactions in response to visible light resulting in the transmission of nerve impulses to the brain. [NIH]

Ribonucleic acid: RNA. One of the two nucleic acids found in all cells. The other is deoxyribonucleic acid (DNA). Ribonucleic acid transfers genetic information from DNA to proteins produced by the cell. [NIH]

Risk factor: A habit, trait, condition, or genetic alteration that increases a person's chance of developing a disease. [NIH]

Rod: A reception for vision, located in the retina. [NIH]

Rubber: A high-molecular-weight polymeric elastomer derived from the milk juice (latex) of Hevea brasiliensis and other trees. It is a substance that can be stretched at room temperature to atleast twice its original length and after releasing the stress, retractrapidly, and recover its original dimensions fully. Synthetic rubber is made from many different chemicals, including styrene, acrylonitrile, ethylene, propylene, and isoprene. [NIH]

Salivary: The duct that convey saliva to the mouth. [NIH]

Salivary glands: Glands in the mouth that produce saliva. [NIH]

Saponins: Sapogenin glycosides. A type of glycoside widely distributed in plants. Each consists of a sapogenin as the aglycon moiety, and a sugar. The sapogenin may be a steroid or a triterpene and the sugar may be glucose, galactose, a pentose, or a methylpentose. Sapogenins are poisonous towards the lower forms of life and are powerful hemolytics when injected into the blood stream able to dissolve red blood cells at even extreme dilutions. [NIH]

Sclerosis: A pathological process consisting of hardening or fibrosis of an anatomical structure, often a vessel or a nerve. [NIH]

Screening: Checking for disease when there are no symptoms. [NIH]

Sebaceous: Gland that secretes sebum. [NIH]

Sebaceous gland: Gland that secretes sebum. [NIH]

Secretion: 1. The process of elaborating a specific product as a result of the activity of a gland; this activity may range from separating a specific substance of the blood to the elaboration of a new chemical substance. 2. Any substance produced by secretion. [EU]

Secretory: Secreting; relating to or influencing secretion or the secretions. [NIH]

Seizures: Clinical or subclinical disturbances of cortical function due to a sudden, abnormal, excessive, and disorganized discharge of brain cells. Clinical manifestations include abnormal motor, sensory and psychic phenomena. Recurrent seizures are usually referred to as epilepsy or "seizure disorder." [NIH]

Semen: The thick, yellowish-white, viscid fluid secretion of male reproductive organs discharged upon ejaculation. In addition to reproductive organ secretions, it contains spermatozoa and their nutrient plasma. [NIH]

Seminiferous tubule: Tube used to transport sperm made in the testes. [NIH]

Semisynthetic: Produced by chemical manipulation of naturally occurring substances. [EU]

Senescence: The bodily and mental state associated with advancing age. [NIH]

Septal: An abscess occurring at the root of the tooth on the proximal surface. [NIH]

Septum: A dividing wall or partition; a general term for such a structure. The term is often used alone to refer to the septal area or to the septum pellucidum. [EU]

Septum Pellucidum: A triangular double membrane separating the anterior horns of the lateral ventricles of the brain. It is situated in the median plane and bounded by the corpus callosum and the body and columns of the fornix. [NIH]

Sequencing: The determination of the order of nucleotides in a DNA or RNA chain. [NIH]

Serine: A non-essential amino acid occurring in natural form as the L-isomer. It is synthesized from glycine or threonine. It is involved in the biosynthesis of purines, pyrimidines, and other amino acids. [NIH]

Serotonin: A biochemical messenger and regulator, synthesized from the essential amino acid L-tryptophan. In humans it is found primarily in the central nervous system, gastrointestinal tract, and blood platelets. Serotonin mediates several important physiological functions including neurotransmission, gastrointestinal motility, hemostasis, and cardiovascular integrity. Multiple receptor families (receptors, serotonin) explain the broad physiological actions and distribution of this biochemical mediator. [NIH]

Serum: The clear liquid part of the blood that remains after blood cells and clotting proteins have been removed. [NIH]

Sex Characteristics: Those characteristics that distinguish one sex from the other. The primary sex characteristics are the ovaries and testes and their related hormones. Secondary sex characteristics are those which are masculine or feminine but not directly related to reproduction. [NIH]

Sex Determination: The biological characteristics which distinguish human beings as female or male. [NIH]

Sex Hormone-Binding Globulin: A glycoprotein migrating as a beta-globulin. Its molecular weight, 52,000 or 95,000-115,000, indicates that it exists as a dimer. The protein binds testosterone, dihydrotestosterone, and estradiol in the plasma. Sex hormone-binding protein has the same amino acid sequence as androgen-binding protein. They differ by their sites of synthesis and post-translational oligosacaccharide modifications. [NIH]

Shivering: Involuntary contraction or twitching of the muscles. It is a physiologic method of heat production in man and other mammals. [NIH]

Signal Transduction: The intercellular or intracellular transfer of information (biological activation/inhibition) through a signal pathway. In each signal transduction system, an activation/inhibition signal from a biologically active molecule (hormone, neurotransmitter) is mediated via the coupling of a receptor/enzyme to a second messenger system or to an ion channel. Signal transduction plays an important role in activating cellular functions, cell differentiation, and cell proliferation. Examples of signal transduction systems are the GABA-postsynaptic receptor-calcium ion channel system, the receptor-mediated T-cell activation pathway, and the receptor-mediated activation of phospholipases. Those coupled to membrane depolarization or intracellular release of calcium include the receptor-mediated activation of cytotoxic functions in granulocytes and the synaptic potentiation of protein kinase activation. Some signal transduction pathways may be part of larger signal transduction pathways; for example, protein kinase activation is part of the platelet activation signal pathway. [NIH]

Skeletal: Having to do with the skeleton (boney part of the body). [NIH]

Skeleton: The framework that supports the soft tissues of vertebrate animals and protects many of their internal organs. The skeletons of vertebrates are made of bone and/or cartilage. [NIH]

Skull: The skeleton of the head including the bones of the face and the bones enclosing the brain. [NIH]

Small intestine: The part of the digestive tract that is located between the stomach and the large intestine. [NIH]

Smooth muscle: Muscle that performs automatic tasks, such as constricting blood vessels. [NIH]

Social Environment: The aggregate of social and cultural institutions, forms, patterns, and processes that influence the life of an individual or community. [NIH]

Sodium: An element that is a member of the alkali group of metals. It has the atomic symbol Na, atomic number 11, and atomic weight 23. With a valence of 1, it has a strong affinity for oxygen and other nonmetallic elements. Sodium provides the chief cation of the extracellular body fluids. Its salts are the most widely used in medicine. (From Dorland, 27th ed) Physiologically the sodium ion plays a major role in blood pressure regulation, maintenance of fluid volume, and electrolyte balance. [NIH]

Sodium Channels: Cell membrane glycoproteins selective for sodium ions. Fast sodium current is associated with the action potential in neural membranes. [NIH]

Somatic: 1. Pertaining to or characteristic of the soma or body. 2. Pertaining to the body wall in contrast to the viscera. [EU]

Somatic cells: All the body cells except the reproductive (germ) cells. [NIH]

Somatostatin: A polypeptide hormone produced in the hypothalamus, and other tissues and organs. It inhibits the release of human growth hormone, and also modulates important physiological functions of the kidney, pancreas, and gastrointestinal tract. Somatostatin receptors are widely expressed throughout the body. Somatostatin also acts as a neurotransmitter in the central and peripheral nervous systems. [NIH]

Sound wave: An alteration of properties of an elastic medium, such as pressure, particle displacement, or density, that propagates through the medium, or a superposition of such alterations. [NIH]

Specialist: In medicine, one who concentrates on 1 special branch of medical science. [NIH]

Species: A taxonomic category subordinate to a genus (or subgenus) and superior to a subspecies or variety, composed of individuals possessing common characters distinguishing them from other categories of individuals of the same taxonomic level. In taxonomic nomenclature, species are designated by the genus name followed by a Latin or Latinized adjective or noun. [EU]

Specificity: Degree of selectivity shown by an antibody with respect to the number and types of antigens with which the antibody combines, as well as with respect to the rates and the extents of these reactions. [NIH]

Spectrum: A charted band of wavelengths of electromagnetic vibrations obtained by refraction and diffraction. By extension, a measurable range of activity, such as the range of bacteria affected by an antibiotic (antibacterial s.) or the complete range of manifestations of a disease. [EU]

Sperm: The fecundating fluid of the male. [NIH]

Spinal cord: The main trunk or bundle of nerves running down the spine through holes in the spinal bone (the vertebrae) from the brain to the level of the lower back. [NIH]

Spontaneous Abortion: The non-induced birth of an embryo or of fetus prior to the stage of viability at about 20 weeks of gestation. [NIH]

Sporadic: Neither endemic nor epidemic; occurring occasionally in a random or isolated manner. [EU]

Steel: A tough, malleable, iron-based alloy containing up to, but no more than, two percent carbon and often other metals. It is used in medicine and dentistry in implants and instrumentation. [NIH]

Sterility: 1. The inability to produce offspring, i.e., the inability to conceive (female s.) or to induce conception (male s.). 2. The state of being aseptic, or free from microorganisms. [EU]

Sterilization: The destroying of all forms of life, especially microorganisms, by heat, chemical, or other means. [NIH]

Steroid: A group name for lipids that contain a hydrogenated cyclopentanoperhydrophenanthrene ring system. Some of the substances included in this group are progesterone, adrenocortical hormones, the gonadal hormones, cardiac aglycones, bile acids, sterols (such as cholesterol), toad poisons, saponins, and some of the carcinogenic hydrocarbons. [EU]

Stillbirth: The birth of a dead fetus or baby. [NIH]

Stimulus: That which can elicit or evoke action (response) in a muscle, nerve, gland or other excitable issue, or cause an augmenting action upon any function or metabolic process. [NIH]

Stomach: An organ of digestion situated in the left upper quadrant of the abdomen between the termination of the esophagus and the beginning of the duodenum. [NIH]

Stool: The waste matter discharged in a bowel movement; feces. [NIH]

Stress: Forcibly exerted influence; pressure. Any condition or situation that causes strain or tension. Stress may be either physical or psychologic, or both. [NIH]

Stroke: Sudden loss of function of part of the brain because of loss of blood flow. Stroke may be caused by a clot (thrombosis) or rupture (hemorrhage) of a blood vessel to the brain. [NIH]

Stroma: The middle, thickest layer of tissue in the cornea. [NIH]

Stromal: Large, veil-like cell in the bone marrow. [NIH]

Stromal Cells: Connective tissue cells of an organ found in the loose connective tissue. These are most often associated with the uterine mucosa and the ovary as well as the hematopoietic system and elsewhere. [NIH]

Subclinical: Without clinical manifestations; said of the early stage(s) of an infection or other disease or abnormality before symptoms and signs become apparent or detectable by clinical examination or laboratory tests, or of a very mild form of an infection or other disease or abnormality. [EU]

Subcutaneous: Beneath the skin. [NIH]

Subspecies: A category intermediate in rank between species and variety, based on a smaller number of correlated characters than are used to differentiate species and generally conditioned by geographical and/or ecological occurrence. [NIH]

Substance P: An eleven-amino acid neurotransmitter that appears in both the central and peripheral nervous systems. It is involved in transmission of pain, causes rapid contractions of the gastrointestinal smooth muscle, and modulates inflammatory and immune responses. [NIH]

Substrate: A substance upon which an enzyme acts. [EU]

Superovulation: Occurrence or induction of release of more ova than are normally released at the same time in a given species. The term applies to both animals and humans. [NIH]

Supplementation: Adding nutrients to the diet. [NIH]

Suppression: A conscious exclusion of disapproved desire contrary with repression, in which the process of exclusion is not conscious. [NIH]

Sympathomimetic: 1. Mimicking the effects of impulses conveyed by adrenergic postganglionic fibres of the sympathetic nervous system. 2. An agent that produces effects similar to those of impulses conveyed by adrenergic postganglionic fibres of the sympathetic nervous system. Called also adrenergic. [EU]

Symphysis: A secondary cartilaginous joint. [NIH]

Symptomatic: Having to do with symptoms, which are signs of a condition or disease. [NIH]

Synapse: The region where the processes of two neurons come into close contiguity, and the nervous impulse passes from one to the other; the fibers of the two are intermeshed, but, according to the general view, there is no direct contiguity. [NIH]

Synapsis: The pairing between homologous chromosomes of maternal and paternal origin during the prophase of meiosis, leading to the formation of gametes. [NIH]

Synaptic: Pertaining to or affecting a synapse (= site of functional apposition between neurons, at which an impulse is transmitted from one neuron to another by electrical or chemical means); pertaining to synapsis (= pairing off in point-for-point association of homologous chromosomes from the male and female pronuclei during the early prophase of meiosis). [EU]

Synchrony: The normal physiologic sequencing of atrial and ventricular activation and contraction. [NIH]

Synergistic: Acting together; enhancing the effect of another force or agent. [EU]

Systemic: Affecting the entire body. [NIH]

Systolic: Indicating the maximum arterial pressure during contraction of the left ventricle of the heart. [EU]

Telangiectasia: The permanent enlargement of blood vessels, causing redness in the skin or mucous membranes. [NIH]

Telencephalon: Paired anteriolateral evaginations of the prosencephalon plus the lamina terminalis. The cerebral hemispheres are derived from it. Many authors consider cerebrum a synonymous term to telencephalon, though a minority include diencephalon as part of the cerebrum (Anthoney, 1994). [NIH]

Temporal: One of the two irregular bones forming part of the lateral surfaces and base of the skull, and containing the organs of hearing. [NIH]

Temporal Lobe: Lower lateral part of the cerebral hemisphere. [NIH]

Teratoma: A type of germ cell tumor that may contain several different types of tissue, such as hair, muscle, and bone. Teratomas occur most often in the ovaries in women, the testicles in men, and the tailbone in children. Not all teratomas are malignant. [NIH]

Testicle: The male gonad where, in adult life, spermatozoa develop; the testis. [NIH]

Testis: Either of the paired male reproductive glands that produce the male germ cells and the male hormones. [NIH]

Testosterone: A hormone that promotes the development and maintenance of male sex characteristics. [NIH]

Thalamic: Cell that reaches the lateral nucleus of amygdala. [NIH]

Thalamic Diseases: Disorders of the centrally located thalamus, which integrates a wide range of cortical and subcortical information. Manifestations include sensory loss, movement disorders; ataxia, pain syndromes, visual disorders, a variety of neuropsychological conditions, and coma. Relatively common etiologies include cerebrovascular disorders; craniocerebral trauma; brain neoplasms; brain hypoxia; intracranial hemorrhages; and infectious processes. [NIH]

Theca Cells: The connective tissue cells of the ovarian follicle. [NIH]

Thermogenesis: The generation of heat in order to maintain body temperature. The uncoupled oxidation of fatty acids contained within brown adipose tissue and shivering are examples of thermogenesis in mammals. [NIH]

Third Ventricle: A narrow cleft inferior to the corpus callosum, within the diencephalon, between the paired thalami. Its floor is formed by the hypothalamus, its anterior wall by the lamina terminalis, and its roof by ependyma. It communicates with the fourth ventricle by the cerebral aqueduct, and with the lateral ventricles by the interventricular foramina. [NIH]

Threshold: For a specified sensory modality (e. g. light, sound, vibration), the lowest level (absolute threshold) or smallest difference (difference threshold, difference limen) or intensity of the stimulus discernible in prescribed conditions of stimulation. [NIH]

Thrombin: An enzyme formed from prothrombin that converts fibrinogen to fibrin.

(Dorland, 27th ed) EC 3.4.21.5. [NIH]

Thrombomodulin: A cell surface glycoprotein of endothelial cells that binds thrombin and serves as a cofactor in the activation of protein C and its regulation of blood coagulation. [NIH]

Thrombophilia: A disorder of hemostasis in which there is a tendency for the occurrence of thrombosis. [NIH]

Thrombosis: The formation or presence of a blood clot inside a blood vessel. [NIH]

Thromboxanes: Physiologically active compounds found in many organs of the body. They are formed in vivo from the prostaglandin endoperoxides and cause platelet aggregation, contraction of arteries, and other biological effects. Thromboxanes are important mediators of the actions of polyunsaturated fatty acids transformed by cyclooxygenase. [NIH]

Thyroid: A gland located near the windpipe (trachea) that produces thyroid hormone, which helps regulate growth and metabolism. [NIH]

Thyrotropin: A peptide hormone secreted by the anterior pituitary. It promotes the growth of the thyroid gland and stimulates the synthesis of thyroid hormones and the release of thyroxine by the thyroid gland. [NIH]

Tissue: A group or layer of cells that are alike in type and work together to perform a specific function. [NIH]

Tissue Plasminogen Activator: A proteolytic enzyme in the serine protease family found in many tissues which converts plasminogen to plasmin. It has fibrin-binding activity and is immunologically different from urinary plasminogen activator. The primary sequence, composed of 527 amino acids, is identical in both the naturally occurring and synthetic proteases. EC 3.4.21.68. [NIH]

Tolerance: 1. The ability to endure unusually large doses of a drug or toxin. 2. Acquired drug tolerance; a decreasing response to repeated constant doses of a drug or the need for increasing doses to maintain a constant response. [EU]

Tomography: Imaging methods that result in sharp images of objects located on a chosen plane and blurred images located above or below the plane. [NIH]

Tone: 1. The normal degree of vigour and tension; in muscle, the resistance to passive elongation or stretch; tonus. 2. A particular quality of sound or of voice. 3. To make permanent, or to change, the colour of silver stain by chemical treatment, usually with a heavy metal. [EU]

Tonus: A state of slight tension usually present in muscles even when they are not undergoing active contraction. [NIH]

Toxaemia: 1. The condition resulting from the spread of bacterial products (toxins) by the bloodstream. 2. A condition resulting from metabolic disturbances, e.g. toxaemia of pregnancy. [EU]

Toxemia: A generalized intoxication produced by toxins and other substances elaborated by an infectious agent. [NIH]

Toxic: Having to do with poison or something harmful to the body. Toxic substances usually cause unwanted side effects. [NIH]

Toxicology: The science concerned with the detection, chemical composition, and pharmacologic action of toxic substances or poisons and the treatment and prevention of toxic manifestations. [NIH]

Toxins: Specific, characterizable, poisonous chemicals, often proteins, with specific biological properties, including immunogenicity, produced by microbes, higher plants, or animals. [NIH]

Trace element: Substance or element essential to plant or animal life, but present in extremely small amounts. [NIH]

Traction: The act of pulling. [NIH]

Transcription Factors: Endogenous substances, usually proteins, which are effective in the initiation, stimulation, or termination of the genetic transcription process. [NIH]

Transduction: The transfer of genes from one cell to another by means of a viral (in the case of bacteria, a bacteriophage) vector or a vector which is similar to a virus particle (pseudovirion). [NIH]

Transfection: The uptake of naked or purified DNA into cells, usually eukaryotic. It is analogous to bacterial transformation. [NIH]

Transgenes: Genes that are introduced into an organism using gene transfer techniques. [NIH]

Translational: The cleavage of signal sequence that directs the passage of the protein through a cell or organelle membrane. [NIH]

Translocation: The movement of material in solution inside the body of the plant. [NIH]

Transmitter: A chemical substance which effects the passage of nerve impulses from one cell to the other at the synapse. [NIH]

Transplantation: Transference of a tissue or organ, alive or dead, within an individual, between individuals of the same species, or between individuals of different species. [NIH]

Treatment Outcome: Evaluation undertaken to assess the results or consequences of management and procedures used in combating disease in order to determine the efficacy, effectiveness, safety, practicability, etc., of these interventions in individual cases or series. [NIH]

Tricuspid Atresia: Absence of the orifice between the right atrium and ventricle, with the presence of an atrial defect through which all the systemic venous return reaches the left heart. As a result, there is left ventricular hypertrophy because the right ventricle is absent or not functional. [NIH]

Triptorelin: A long-acting gonadorelin analog agonist. It has been used in the treatment of prostatic cancer, ovarian cancer, precocious puberty, endometriosis, and to induce ovulation for in vitro fertilization. [NIH]

Troglitazone: A drug used in diabetes treatment that is being studied for its effect on reducing the risk of cancer cell growth in fat tissue. [NIH]

Trophic: Of or pertaining to nutrition. [EU]

Trophoblast: The outer layer of cells of the blastocyst which works its way into the endometrium during ovum implantation and grows rapidly, later combining with mesoderm. [NIH]

Tuberous Sclerosis: A rare congenital disease in which the essential pathology is the appearance of multiple tumors in the cerebrum and in other organs, such as the heart or kidneys. [NIH]

Tumor marker: A substance sometimes found in an increased amount in the blood, other body fluids, or tissues and which may mean that a certain type of cancer is in the body. Examples of tumor markers include CA 125 (ovarian cancer), CA 15-3 (breast cancer), CEA (ovarian, lung, breast, pancreas, and gastrointestinal tract cancers), and PSA (prostate cancer). Also called biomarker. [NIH]

Type 2 diabetes: Usually characterized by a gradual onset with minimal or no symptoms of metabolic disturbance and no requirement for exogenous insulin. The peak age of onset is 50 to 60 years. Obesity and possibly a genetic factor are usually present. [NIH]

Tyrosine: A non-essential amino acid. In animals it is synthesized from phenylalanine. It is also the precursor of epinephrine, thyroid hormones, and melanin. [NIH]

Ultrasonography: The visualization of deep structures of the body by recording the reflections of echoes of pulses of ultrasonic waves directed into the tissues. Use of ultrasound for imaging or diagnostic purposes employs frequencies ranging from 1.6 to 10 megahertz. [NIH]

Unconscious: Experience which was once conscious, but was subsequently rejected, as the "personal unconscious". [NIH]

Urethra: The tube through which urine leaves the body. It empties urine from the bladder. [NIH]

Urinary: Having to do with urine or the organs of the body that produce and get rid of urine. [NIH]

Urinary Plasminogen Activator: A proteolytic enzyme that converts plasminogen to plasmin where the preferential cleavage is between arginine and valine. It was isolated originally from human urine, but is found in most tissues of most vertebrates. EC 3.4.21.73. [NIH]

Urine: Fluid containing water and waste products. Urine is made by the kidneys, stored in the bladder, and leaves the body through the urethra. [NIH]

Uterus: The small, hollow, pear-shaped organ in a woman's pelvis. This is the organ in which a fetus develops. Also called the womb. [NIH]

Vaccine: A substance or group of substances meant to cause the immune system to respond to a tumor or to microorganisms, such as bacteria or viruses. [NIH]

Vagina: The muscular canal extending from the uterus to the exterior of the body. Also called the birth canal. [NIH]

Vaginal: Of or having to do with the vagina, the birth canal. [NIH]

Valproic Acid: A fatty acid with anticonvulsant properties used in the treatment of epilepsy. The mechanisms of its therapeutic actions are not well understood. It may act by increasing GABA levels in the brain or by altering the properties of voltage dependent sodium channels. [NIH]

Vascular: Pertaining to blood vessels or indicative of a copious blood supply. [EU]

Vasodilation: Physiological dilation of the blood vessels without anatomic change. For dilation with anatomic change, dilatation, pathologic or aneurysm (or specific aneurysm) is used. [NIH]

Vasodilator: An agent that widens blood vessels. [NIH]

Vein: Vessel-carrying blood from various parts of the body to the heart. [NIH]

Venous: Of or pertaining to the veins. [EU]

Ventricle: One of the two pumping chambers of the heart. The right ventricle receives oxygen-poor blood from the right atrium and pumps it to the lungs through the pulmonary artery. The left ventricle receives oxygen-rich blood from the left atrium and pumps it to the body through the aorta. [NIH]

Ventricular: Pertaining to a ventricle. [EU]

Vesicular: 1. Composed of or relating to small, saclike bodies. 2. Pertaining to or made up of vesicles on the skin. [EU]

Veterinary Medicine: The medical science concerned with the prevention, diagnosis, and treatment of diseases in animals. [NIH]

Vinyl Chloride: A gas that has been used as an aerosol propellant and is the starting material for polyvinyl resins. Toxicity studies have shown various adverse effects, particularly the occurrence of liver neoplasms. [NIH]

Virilism: Development of masculine traits in the female. [NIH]

Virilization: The induction or development of male secondary sec characters, especially the induction of such changes in the female, including enlargement of the clitoris, growth of facial and body hair, development of a hairline typical of the male forehead, stimulation of secretion and proliferation of the sebaceous glands (often with acne), and deepening of the voice. Called also masculinization) [EU]

Virus: Submicroscopic organism that causes infectious disease. In cancer therapy, some viruses may be made into vaccines that help the body build an immune response to, and kill, tumor cells. [NIH]

Vitamin A: A substance used in cancer prevention; it belongs to the family of drugs called retinoids. [NIH]

Vitro: Descriptive of an event or enzyme reaction under experimental investigation occurring outside a living organism. Parts of an organism or microorganism are used together with artificial substrates and/or conditions. [NIH]

Vivo: Outside of or removed from the body of a living organism. [NIH]

White blood cell: A type of cell in the immune system that helps the body fight infection and disease. White blood cells include lymphocytes, granulocytes, macrophages, and others. [NIH]

Womb: A hollow, thick-walled, muscular organ in which the impregnated ovum is developed into a child. [NIH]

Xenograft: The cells of one species transplanted to another species. [NIH]

X-ray: High-energy radiation used in low doses to diagnose diseases and in high doses to treat cancer. [NIH]

Yeasts: A general term for single-celled rounded fungi that reproduce by budding. Brewers' and bakers' yeasts are Saccharomyces cerevisiae; therapeutic dried yeast is dried yeast. [NIH]

Zona Pellucida: The transport non-cellular envelope surrounding the mammalian ovum. [NIH]

Zygote: The fertilized ovum. [NIH]

Zymogen: Inactive form of an enzyme which can then be converted to the active form, usually by excision of a polypeptide, e. g. trypsinogen is the zymogen of trypsin. [NIH]

INDEX

A

Abdomen, 135, 141, 160, 161, 167, 174, 178
Abdominal, 96, 135, 167, 170, 174
Aberrant, 9, 135
Ablation, 135, 137
Abortion, 135, 170
Acanthosis Nigricans, 4, 5, 88, 89, 135
Acetylcholine, 135, 165
Acne, 88, 92, 96, 135, 148, 183
Acrylonitrile, 18, 135, 175
Adaptability, 135, 142, 143
Adenovirus, 14, 26, 135
Adhesions, 56, 135
Adhesives, 135
Adipocytes, 135, 146, 160
Adipose Tissue, 135, 179
Adjuvant, 79, 135
Adolescence, 22, 136
Adrenal Cortex, 93, 136, 137, 147, 152, 156, 171, 173
Adrenal Glands, 93, 136
Adrenal Medulla, 136, 142, 152, 165
Adrenergic, 136, 150, 152, 178
Adverse Effect, 136, 168, 183
Aerosol, 136, 183
Afferent, 136, 160
Affinity, 95, 136, 176
Agar, 136, 169
Age of Onset, 136, 182
Agonist, 30, 37, 40, 41, 63, 70, 71, 95, 96, 136, 144, 150, 161, 164, 181
Algorithms, 136, 140
Alkaline, 136, 141
Alleles, 136, 156
Allergen, 136, 149
Alternative medicine, 106, 136
Alveoli, 137, 148
Amenorrhea, 40, 65, 84, 92, 131, 137, 169
Amino acid, 137, 138, 140, 150, 154, 160, 163, 165, 168, 172, 175, 176, 178, 180, 182
Amino Acid Sequence, 137, 140, 176
Amplification, 14, 137
Anabolic, 17, 137, 149
Anaesthesia, 137, 158
Analog, 62, 71, 137, 160, 181
Analogous, 137, 181
Anatomical, 23, 137, 139, 143, 149, 158, 175
Androgen suppression, 89, 137

Androgen-Binding Protein, 137, 176
Androgenic, 17, 66, 93, 137
Androgens, 6, 7, 9, 12, 15, 23, 25, 31, 35, 42, 48, 49, 65, 88, 100, 136, 137, 147, 156
Androstenedione, 10, 18, 35, 74, 137
Anemia, 117, 137
Aneurysm, 137, 182
Angiography, 54, 137
Angiotensinogen, 138, 173
Animal model, 101, 138
Anovulation, 7, 8, 9, 13, 15, 18, 22, 25, 40, 67, 80, 92, 138, 169
Antibacterial, 138, 177
Antibiotic, 138, 141, 177
Antibody, 136, 138, 145, 151, 155, 156, 157, 158, 162, 177
Anticoagulant, 138, 172
Anticonvulsant, 138, 141, 168, 182
Antiemetic, 138, 150, 163
Antiepileptic, 13, 55, 138
Antifungal, 138, 159
Antigen, 29, 136, 138, 145, 152, 156, 157, 158, 162
Anti-inflammatory, 138, 147, 149, 154
Anti-Inflammatory Agents, 138, 147
Antineoplastic, 138, 147
Anus, 138, 139, 141, 144, 159
Apolipoproteins, 138, 161
Apoptosis, 14, 138, 142
Arachidonic Acid, 81, 139, 160, 171
Arterial, 76, 139, 143, 146, 157, 172, 179
Arteries, 139, 141, 147, 161, 163, 172, 180
Arteriolar, 139, 173
Arteriosclerosis, 88, 139, 157, 174
Artery, 7, 88, 137, 139, 147, 172
Arthrosis, 139, 162
Assay, 8, 26, 139, 157
Asymptomatic, 4, 139
Ataxia, 116, 117, 139, 179
Atresia, 15, 24, 139
Atrial, 139, 146, 179, 181
Atrioventricular, 139, 146
Atrium, 139, 146, 181, 182
Atrophy, 116, 139
Axillary, 139, 141
Axillary Artery, 139, 141

B

Bacteria, 138, 139, 140, 152, 163, 177, 181, 182
Bacteriophage, 139, 169, 181
Bacterium, 140, 145
Basal Ganglia, 139, 140
Basal Ganglia Diseases, 139, 140
Base, 140, 148, 159, 179
Benign, 95, 140, 155
Beta-Endorphin, 59, 140
Bilateral, 140, 169
Bile, 140, 153, 161, 177
Biochemical, 7, 10, 14, 66, 136, 140, 175
Biomarkers, 9, 140
Biotechnology, 26, 27, 100, 106, 113, 115, 116, 117, 140
Bipolar Disorder, 28, 68, 73, 140
Bladder, 66, 140, 145, 171, 182
Blastocyst, 12, 20, 140, 145, 151, 167, 169, 181
Blood Coagulation, 140, 141, 180
Blood Glucose, 4, 5, 140, 155, 159
Blood pressure, 10, 96, 140, 142, 157, 163, 172, 176
Blood vessel, 137, 140, 141, 142, 143, 144, 146, 159, 176, 178, 179, 180, 182
Blot, 19, 141
Body Fluids, 140, 141, 176, 181
Body Mass Index, 31, 63, 141, 167
Bolus, 51, 141
Bolus infusion, 141
Bone Marrow, 141, 153, 178
Bowel, 141, 149, 178
Bowel Movement, 141, 149, 178
Brachial, 88, 141
Brachial Artery, 88, 141
Branch, 24, 129, 141, 150, 167, 172, 177
Broad-spectrum, 22, 141

C

Calcium, 7, 23, 49, 68, 76, 77, 92, 141, 145, 176
Calcium channel blocker, 49, 141
Calcium Channel Blockers, 49, 141
Caloric intake, 4, 141
Carbamazepine, 74, 141
Carbohydrate, 94, 142, 147, 154, 169
Carbon Dioxide, 142, 169, 174
Carcinogenic, 142, 158, 171, 177
Carcinogens, 142, 143, 166
Carcinoma, 38, 66, 142, 148
Cardiac, 30, 142, 146, 152, 164, 177
Cardiovascular, 7, 10, 21, 22, 32, 88, 97, 142, 160, 174, 176
Cardiovascular disease, 10, 21, 22, 97, 142, 174
Carotene, 142, 174
Case report, 34, 50, 58, 61, 79, 142
Caspase, 14, 142
Castration, 142
Catecholamine, 48, 142, 150
Caudal, 142, 149, 157, 170
Causal, 25, 142
Caveolins, 142, 144
Cell Aggregation, 142, 166
Cell Death, 138, 142
Cell Differentiation, 14, 142, 176
Cell Division, 116, 139, 143, 162, 163, 169, 171
Cell membrane, 15, 141, 143, 148, 168, 177
Cell proliferation, 24, 43, 139, 143, 176
Cell Survival, 14, 24, 143
Cerebellar, 139, 143, 173
Cerebral, 13, 139, 140, 143, 146, 152, 172, 179
Cerebral Cortex, 13, 139, 143
Cerebrovascular, 140, 141, 142, 143, 179
Cerebrum, 143, 179, 181
Cervical, 12, 143
Cervix, 135, 143, 174
Chemotaxis, 12, 143
Chin, 43, 72, 81, 82, 143, 162
Cholesterol, 19, 84, 140, 143, 144, 147, 150, 156, 161, 177
Cholesterol Esters, 143, 161
Chromaffin System, 143, 151
Chromatin, 138, 143
Chromium, 96, 143
Chromosomal, 24, 62, 137, 143
Chromosome, 143, 160
Chronic, 8, 11, 15, 22, 25, 29, 47, 92, 93, 94, 116, 144, 149, 151, 158, 159, 160, 169
Chronic Disease, 144, 160
Chronic renal, 144, 169
Chylomicrons, 144, 161
Circulatory system, 144, 151
CIS, 17, 24, 26, 144, 174
Clamp, 21, 144
Clathrin, 16, 144, 151
Clathrin-Coated Vesicles, 16, 144
Clinical trial, 6, 87, 89, 95, 113, 144, 146, 173
Clomiphene, 8, 34, 40, 55, 56, 58, 61, 64, 66, 67, 70, 72, 74, 87, 89, 93, 144

Clone, 16, 24, 144
Cloning, 140, 144
Coated Vesicles, 16, 144, 151
Cofactor, 144, 172, 180
Colon, 96, 116, 144, 160
Competency, 20, 145
Complement, 145, 161, 169
Complementary and alternative
    medicine, 79, 84, 145
Complementary medicine, 79, 145
Compliance, 22, 145
Computational Biology, 113, 115, 145
Computed tomography, 65, 145
Computerized tomography, 145
Conception, 12, 42, 72, 95, 135, 145, 146,
    153, 170, 177
Cones, 146, 174
Conjugated, 146, 148
Connective Tissue, 141, 146, 153, 161, 178,
    179
Connective Tissue Cells, 146, 179
Contraception, 43, 95, 146
Contraceptive Agents, 95, 146
Contraindications, ii, 146
Contrast medium, 137, 146
Control group, 14, 146
Controlled study, 34, 56, 70, 146
Conventional therapy, 146
Conventional treatment, 71, 146
Convulsions, 138, 146, 150, 170
Coordination, 12, 146
Cor, 6, 51, 74, 80, 146, 147
Cornea, 147, 178
Coronary, 7, 88, 101, 142, 147, 163
Coronary heart disease, 101, 142, 147
Coronary Thrombosis, 147, 163
Corpus, 147, 161, 167, 171, 175, 179
Corpus Luteum, 147, 161, 171
Cortex, 147, 173
Cortical, 147, 175, 179
Corticosteroid, 6, 147
Corticotropin-Releasing Hormone, 51, 74,
    147
Cortisol, 24, 147
Cortisone, 147, 149
Cost-benefit, 75, 147
Cost-Benefit Analysis, 75, 147
Cyclic, 19, 147, 171
Cyclin, 19, 148
Cyclin-Dependent Kinases, 19, 148
Cyproterone, 34, 37, 148, 153
Cyproterone Acetate, 34, 37, 148

Cyst, 148, 167
Cytochrome, 13, 36, 148
Cytoplasm, 138, 143, 148, 155, 173
Cytotoxic, 148, 176

D

Decidua, 148, 169
Dehydroepiandrosterone, 93, 148
Deletion, 138, 148
Dendrites, 148, 165
Density, 17, 141, 148, 150, 161, 166, 177
Dentition, 50, 148
Deoxyribonucleic, 148, 174
Deoxyribonucleic acid, 148, 174
Depolarization, 148, 176
Depressive Disorder, 34, 149
Desensitization, 37, 149
Dexamethasone, 6, 71, 149
Diabetes Insipidus, 149, 169
Diabetes Mellitus, 9, 11, 16, 21, 56, 58, 84,
    94, 96, 97, 101, 149, 154, 155, 169, 174
Diabetic Ketoacidosis, 149, 159
Diagnostic procedure, 91, 106, 149
Diastolic, 149, 157
Diathermy, 33, 36, 43, 46, 47, 48, 149
Diencephalon, 149, 157, 179
Digestion, 140, 141, 149, 161, 178
Digestive system, 90, 149
Dihydrotestosterone, 148, 149, 173, 176
Dilatation, 135, 137, 149, 182
Dilatation, Pathologic, 149, 182
Dilation, 149, 182
Dimerization, 24, 149
Direct, iii, 17, 19, 23, 149, 150, 173, 178
Discrete, 17, 25, 149
Dissociation, 136, 149
Domperidone, 62, 150
Dopa, 41, 150, 160
Dopamine, 32, 62, 150, 160, 163, 165
Dopamine Agonists, 32, 150
Drive, ii, vi, 5, 16, 21, 23, 25, 69, 150, 160
Dyslipidemia, 5, 150
Dysphoric, 149, 150
Dysplasia, 117, 150
Dystrophy, 116, 150

E

Eclampsia, 150, 170
Edema, 150, 167, 170
Effector, 16, 135, 145, 150
Efficacy, 7, 23, 37, 95, 150, 181
Elective, 12, 150
Electrolyte, 147, 150, 163, 170, 177
Electrophysiological, 23, 150

Embryo, 36, 38, 41, 55, 66, 82, 135, 140, 142, 151, 158, 162, 164, 170, 177
Embryo Transfer, 36, 38, 41, 55, 66, 82, 151, 170
Encapsulated, 18, 151
Endocrine Glands, 151, 156
Endocrine System, 17, 151, 165
Endogenous, 140, 150, 151, 181
Endometrial, 9, 12, 20, 38, 151, 167
Endometriosis, 8, 95, 151, 181
Endometrium, 9, 81, 148, 151, 162, 165, 181
Endorphins, 151, 165
Endosomes, 144, 151
End-stage renal, 144, 151, 169
Energy balance, 151, 160
Enkephalin, 140, 151
Environmental Exposure, 151, 166
Environmental Health, 112, 114, 151
Enzymatic, 137, 141, 142, 145, 148, 151, 174
Enzyme, 13, 17, 58, 142, 150, 151, 153, 156, 163, 169, 172, 173, 176, 178, 179, 180, 182, 183
Enzyme-Linked Immunosorbent Assay, 58, 151
Epinephrine, 136, 150, 152, 165, 182
Epithelial, 9, 148, 152
Epithelial Cells, 152
Epithelium, 9, 12, 152
Erythrocytes, 44, 137, 141, 152
Esophagus, 139, 149, 152, 178
Essential Tremor, 116, 152
Estradiol, 18, 23, 25, 30, 39, 54, 64, 152, 176
Estrogen, 9, 17, 21, 24, 39, 144, 148, 152, 161, 171
Estrogen receptor, 17, 39, 144, 152
Ethinyl Estradiol, 34, 152
Excitation, 152, 165
Exogenous, 14, 68, 151, 152, 182
Extrapyramidal, 150, 152
Eye Infections, 135, 152

F

Facial, 88, 152, 183
Fallopian tube, 152, 174
Family Planning, 113, 152
Fat, 4, 16, 31, 48, 101, 135, 139, 141, 142, 146, 147, 152, 159, 160, 161, 167, 181
Fatty acids, 149, 152, 171, 179, 180
Fertilization in Vitro, 152, 170
Fetus, 25, 135, 153, 169, 170, 177, 178, 182
Fibrin, 140, 153, 169, 179, 180
Fibrosis, 117, 153, 175

Flutamide, 54, 153
Fold, 21, 153
Follicles, 14, 18, 24, 64, 153, 158
Follicular Fluid, 56, 153
Follicular Phase, 23, 30, 48, 50, 153
Forearm, 141, 153

G

Gallbladder, 135, 149, 153
Ganglia, 135, 140, 153, 165, 168
Gas, 142, 153, 156, 165, 183
Gastrin, 153, 156
Gastrointestinal, 150, 152, 153, 160, 175, 177, 178, 181
Gastrointestinal tract, 153, 160, 175, 177, 181
Gene, 7, 9, 14, 17, 19, 24, 26, 45, 48, 81, 85, 97, 100, 117, 118, 135, 136, 140, 153, 166, 181
Gene Expression, 7, 9, 25, 26, 97, 117, 153
Gene Therapy, 135, 153
Generator, 7, 54, 153
Genotype, 153, 168
Germ Cells, 11, 153, 162, 166, 167, 179
Gestation, 10, 20, 25, 153, 169, 177
Gestational, 56, 94, 101, 154
Gland, 136, 143, 147, 154, 156, 161, 167, 168, 171, 175, 178, 180
Glucocorticoid, 149, 154
Gluconeogenesis, 96, 154
Glucose Intolerance, 15, 101, 149, 154
Glucose tolerance, 6, 15, 35, 58, 61, 101, 154
Glucose Tolerance Test, 35, 61, 154
Glutamic Acid, 154, 165
Glycine, 137, 154, 165, 175
Glycoprotein, 154, 164, 176, 180
Glycosuria, 4, 94, 154
Gonad, 24, 154, 179
Gonadal, 13, 24, 26, 48, 154, 177
Gonadorelin, 154, 160, 181
Gonadotropic, 23, 25, 154
Gonadotropin, 7, 13, 15, 22, 25, 28, 31, 32, 33, 34, 40, 41, 47, 48, 50, 51, 54, 55, 61, 62, 63, 66, 67, 70, 71, 72, 74, 92, 154, 160
Governing Board, 155, 170
Grade, 47, 155
Graft, 18, 155, 157
Grafting, 18, 155, 158
Granulocytes, 155, 160, 176, 183
Granulosa Cells, 13, 15, 19, 155, 158, 161

H

Haplotypes, 7, 155

Haptens, 136, 155
Headache, 155, 170
Heart attack, 142, 155
Heme, 148, 155
Hemoglobin, 5, 137, 152, 155, 160
Hemoglobinuria, 116, 155
Hemorrhage, 155, 178
Hemostasis, 155, 176, 180
Hepatic, 13, 154, 155
Hereditary, 4, 155, 174
Heredity, 153, 156
Heterogeneity, 136, 156
Heterozygotes, 6, 156
Hirsutism, 7, 22, 92, 131, 148, 156, 157
Homeostasis, 16, 156
Homologous, 136, 153, 156, 178, 179
Hormonal, 21, 25, 31, 42, 45, 76, 93, 139, 147, 156
Hormone Antagonists, 75, 156
Hormone therapy, 31, 57, 61, 156
Horseradish Peroxidase, 152, 156
Hybrid, 144, 156
Hydrogen, 140, 142, 156, 163, 167
Hydrophobic, 156, 160
Hyperandrogenism, 7, 10, 15, 18, 20, 25, 29, 36, 37, 65, 76, 85, 88, 89, 156
Hypercholesterolemia, 84, 150, 156
Hyperglycemia, 4, 5, 94, 96, 156
Hyperlipidemia, 150, 156
Hyperplasia, 18, 49, 156
Hypersecretion, 10, 16, 25, 28, 157
Hypersensitivity, 136, 149, 157, 160
Hyperstimulation, 33, 50, 73, 81, 157
Hypertension, 5, 21, 96, 141, 142, 155, 157, 170, 174
Hyperthermia, 149, 157
Hypertrichosis, 156, 157
Hypertriglyceridemia, 150, 157
Hypertrophy, 147, 157, 181
Hypogonadism, 26, 55, 157
Hypothalamic, 10, 13, 23, 26, 48, 79, 97, 157
Hypothalamus, 13, 17, 21, 147, 149, 151, 154, 157, 168, 170, 177, 179
Hypothyroidism, 4, 157

I
Id, 48, 77, 83, 120, 121, 123, 128, 130, 157
Idiopathic, 13, 157
Immune response, 135, 138, 147, 155, 157, 161, 178, 183
Immunoassay, 151, 157
Immunodeficiency, 116, 157

Immunology, 135, 136, 156, 157
Immunotherapy, 149, 157
Impairment, 16, 18, 139, 152, 158, 162
Implantation, 9, 12, 18, 145, 158, 165, 167
In situ, 17, 19, 158
In vivo, 9, 14, 16, 19, 20, 21, 23, 26, 81, 95, 153, 158, 180
Incision, 158, 159, 160
Indicative, 10, 99, 158, 167, 182
Induction, 19, 44, 48, 51, 72, 74, 81, 137, 149, 158, 167, 171, 178, 183
Infarction, 147, 158, 163
Infection, 152, 157, 158, 161, 178, 183
Inflammation, 47, 135, 138, 152, 153, 158, 160, 169
Infusion, 51, 158
Ingestion, 154, 158
Inhibin, 33, 39, 44, 48, 58, 72, 158
Initiation, 23, 158, 181
Inositol, 15, 97, 158
Inotropic, 150, 158
Insight, 11, 14, 20, 26, 158
Insomnia, 159, 170
Insulin-dependent diabetes mellitus, 159
Insulin-like, 19, 34, 36, 44, 57, 65, 73, 93, 159
Internal Medicine, 7, 15, 72, 73, 74, 151, 159
Interstitial, 18, 21, 159
Intestinal, 142, 154, 159, 161
Intestines, 135, 139, 153, 159
Intoxication, 159, 180
Intracellular, 14, 15, 16, 17, 24, 141, 144, 158, 159, 170, 171, 176
Intravascular, 159, 167
Intravenous, 51, 70, 158, 159
Intrinsic, 21, 136, 159
Invasive, 159, 161
Involuntary, 140, 152, 159, 164, 176
Ischemia, 139, 159

J
Joint, 35, 139, 159, 178

K
Kb, 112, 159
Ketoconazole, 70, 159
Ketone Bodies, 149, 159
Ketonuria, 4, 159
Kidney Disease, 52, 90, 112, 117, 120, 159

L
Lactation, 159, 171
Laparotomy, 18, 160
Large Intestine, 149, 159, 160, 173, 176

Leptin, 35, 56, 60, 160
Lethargy, 157, 160
Leucine, 140, 160
Leucocyte, 160
Leukaemia, 40, 160
Leukemia, 24, 116, 153, 160
Leukotrienes, 81, 139, 160
Leuprolide, 16, 88, 89, 160
Levodopa, 150, 160
Libido, 17, 93, 137, 160
Library Services, 128, 160
Ligament, 152, 160, 172
Ligands, 9, 160
Linkage, 27, 93, 160
Lipid, 34, 96, 138, 139, 159, 160
Lipoprotein, 17, 34, 150, 160, 161
Liposarcoma, 96, 161
Liver, 93, 101, 135, 139, 140, 149, 153, 154, 155, 161, 173, 183
Liver Neoplasms, 161, 183
Lobe, 13, 62, 161
Localization, 11, 13, 161
Localized, 151, 156, 157, 158, 161, 169
Low-density lipoprotein, 150, 161
Luteal Phase, 13, 161
Lutein Cells, 161, 171
Luteinizing hormone-releasing hormone agonist, 29, 161
Lymph, 139, 143, 144, 161
Lymph node, 139, 143, 161
Lymphocyte, 138, 161, 162
Lymphoid, 160, 161
Lymphoma, 116, 161

M

Magnetic Resonance Imaging, 31, 161
Major Histocompatibility Complex, 155, 161
Malabsorption, 116, 161
Malignancy, 135, 162
Malignant, 116, 138, 162, 179
Malnutrition, 139, 162, 164
Manic, 140, 162
McMaster, 72, 74, 162
Medial, 88, 139, 162, 166
Mediate, 16, 17, 19, 26, 150, 162
Mediator, 15, 150, 162, 176
Medical castration, 65, 162
Medical Records, 162, 174
MEDLINE, 113, 115, 117, 162
Meiosis, 162, 178, 179
Melanocytes, 162
Melanoma, 116, 162

Melanosis, 135, 162
Membrane, 143, 144, 145, 148, 151, 162, 164, 166, 168, 170, 174, 175, 176, 181
Menopause, 21, 162
Menstrual Cycle, 9, 10, 20, 21, 23, 50, 60, 95, 153, 161, 162, 170, 171
Menstruation, 120, 137, 148, 153, 161, 162, 166, 170
Mental, iv, 5, 90, 112, 114, 118, 143, 149, 157, 162, 166, 172, 175
Mental Disorders, 90, 162
Mental Health, iv, 5, 90, 112, 114, 162, 166, 172
Mesoderm, 162, 181
Meta-Analysis, 27, 163
Metabolic disorder, 4, 20, 93, 149, 163
Metaphase, 20, 163
Methionine, 140, 163
Metoclopramide, 63, 163
MI, 49, 94, 132, 163
Microorganism, 144, 163, 183
Migration, 18, 163
Mineralocorticoids, 136, 147, 163
Miscarriage, 9, 20, 41, 121, 122, 163
Mitosis, 14, 138, 163
Mobility, 26, 163
Modeling, 21, 163
Modification, 4, 22, 101, 137, 163, 172
Molecular, 8, 12, 16, 18, 19, 26, 27, 48, 113, 115, 140, 145, 163, 169, 171, 175, 176
Molecule, 138, 140, 145, 148, 149, 150, 152, 163, 167, 173, 176
Monitor, 96, 163, 165
Monocyte, 12, 163
Monotherapy, 13, 163
Morphological, 10, 92, 151, 162, 163
Morphology, 13, 18, 25, 50, 67, 74, 80, 163
Morula, 140, 164
Mucolytic, 96, 164
Mucosa, 164, 171, 178
Mucus, 164
Muscle Fibers, 164
Muscular Atrophy, 116, 164
Muscular Dystrophies, 150, 164
Myocardium, 163, 164
Myotonic Dystrophy, 116, 164

N

Naloxone, 140, 164
Naltrexone, 47, 57, 73, 164
Narcotic, 164
Nausea, 138, 164, 170
NCI, 1, 89, 111, 144, 164

Need, 3, 4, 100, 124, 144, 164, 180
Neonatal, 10, 14, 164
Neoplasia, 116, 164
Neoplastic, 161, 164
Nephropathy, 159, 164
Nerve, 80, 136, 139, 143, 148, 162, 164, 165, 166, 170, 174, 175, 178, 181
Nerve Growth Factor, 80, 165
Nervous System, 17, 24, 116, 135, 136, 153, 154, 155, 160, 162, 164, 165, 166, 168, 175, 178
Neural, 17, 23, 136, 165, 177
Neural Pathways, 23, 165
Neuroendocrine, 17, 21, 49, 97, 165
Neuronal, 23, 165
Neurons, 22, 148, 153, 160, 165, 178, 179
Neuropeptide, 147, 165
Neurosecretory Systems, 151, 165
Neurotransmitter, 23, 135, 137, 150, 154, 165, 176, 177, 178
Nidation, 151, 165
Nitrogen, 137, 165
Norepinephrine, 136, 150, 165
Nuclear, 24, 96, 140, 165
Nuclei, 153, 161, 163, 165, 166
Nucleic acid, 165, 174
Nucleus, 138, 140, 143, 147, 148, 162, 166, 171, 173, 179
Nurse Practitioners, 5, 166

O

Occupational Health, 53, 166
Occupational Health Nursing, 53, 166
Oestradiol, 37, 166
Oligo, 92, 166
Oligomenorrhea, 166, 169
Oncogene, 116, 166
Only Child, 4, 166
Oocytes, 20, 56, 61, 62, 73, 74, 166
Opacity, 148, 166
Ophthalmic, 166, 174
Opiate, 23, 140, 151, 164, 166
Opium, 166
Opsin, 166, 174
Optic Chiasm, 157, 166, 170
Optic Nerve, 166, 174
Organelles, 144, 148, 162, 166
Ovarian Cysts, 38, 71, 120, 166
Ovarian Follicle, 19, 21, 23, 39, 147, 153, 155, 166, 179
Ovarian Hyperstimulation Syndrome, 47, 167
Overweight, 4, 22, 77, 97, 101, 167

Ovulation Induction, 30, 37, 56, 60, 68, 72, 73, 74, 75, 167
Ovum, 147, 148, 153, 154, 164, 166, 167, 171, 181, 183
Ovum Implantation, 167, 181
Oxidation, 148, 149, 167, 179

P

Palliative, 148, 167
Pancreas, 135, 140, 149, 159, 167, 177, 181
Pancreatic, 10, 116, 167
Pancreatic cancer, 116, 167
Paroxysmal, 116, 167
Parturition, 167, 171
Pathogenesis, 15, 21, 62, 65, 167
Pathologic, 138, 147, 157, 167
Pathologic Processes, 138, 167
Pathophysiology, 4, 11, 16, 22, 26, 167
Pelvic, 151, 167, 171
Pelvis, 121, 135, 167, 182
Penis, 167, 174
Peptide, 23, 35, 72, 137, 140, 160, 168, 172, 180
Peripheral Nervous System, 165, 168, 177, 178
Peristalsis, 150, 168
Pharmacologic, 5, 70, 168, 180
Phenotype, 10, 14, 39, 168
Phenyl, 95, 168
Phenytoin, 141, 168
Phospholipases, 168, 176
Phospholipids, 152, 158, 161, 168
Phosphorus, 141, 168
Phosphorylated, 15, 168
Phosphorylation, 14, 19, 27, 148, 168
Physical Examination, 4, 11, 168
Physiologic, 26, 70, 136, 150, 162, 168, 171, 173, 176, 179
Physiology, 12, 13, 17, 23, 26, 150, 151, 168
Pigments, 142, 168, 174
Pilot study, 28, 168
Pituitary Gland, 147, 154, 168
Placenta, 93, 152, 169, 171
Plants, 142, 154, 163, 165, 168, 169, 175, 180
Plaque, 88, 169
Plasma, 4, 143, 153, 154, 155, 163, 169, 173, 175, 176
Plasma protein, 153, 169
Plasmin, 169, 180, 182
Plasminogen, 169, 180, 182
Platelet Activation, 169, 176
Pneumonia, 146, 169

Polydipsia, 4, 5, 169
Polymorphism, 45, 81, 169
Polyphagia, 5, 169
Polysaccharide, 138, 169
Polyuria, 4, 5, 169
Posterior, 139, 167, 169
Postnatal, 25, 170
Postprandial, 59, 170
Postsynaptic, 170, 176
Post-translational, 26, 137, 170, 176
Potassium, 23, 163, 170
Potentiation, 170, 176
Practicability, 170, 181
Practice Guidelines, 114, 170
Preclinical, 95, 170
Precursor, 137, 138, 139, 150, 151, 160, 165, 169, 170, 182
Preeclampsia, 13, 170
Pregnancy Complications, 13, 170
Pregnancy Outcome, 30, 55, 170
Premenstrual, 95, 120, 170
Premenstrual Syndrome, 95, 120, 170
Prenatal, 10, 20, 25, 48, 151, 170
Preoptic Area, 17, 170
Presynaptic, 165, 170
Prevalence, 3, 4, 56, 75, 88, 170
Progesterone, 9, 11, 12, 18, 23, 45, 54, 68, 95, 171, 177
Progestogen, 95, 171
Progression, 11, 19, 96, 138, 148, 171
Progressive, 142, 144, 155, 164, 169, 171
Prolactin, 57, 61, 62, 150, 171
Promoter, 15, 17, 19, 26, 171
Prophase, 166, 171, 178, 179
Proportional, 152, 171
Prospective study, 63, 73, 171
Prostaglandin, 81, 171, 180
Prostaglandins A, 171
Prostate, 96, 116, 140, 171, 174, 181
Protease, 172, 180
Protective Agents, 141, 172
Protein C, 42, 137, 138, 139, 144, 160, 172
Protein S, 100, 117, 140, 172
Proteinuria, 170, 172
Proteolytic, 145, 169, 172, 180, 182
Psychic, 160, 162, 172, 175
Psychomotor, 5, 141, 172
Puberty, 4, 17, 22, 26, 57, 172, 181
Public Health, 8, 12, 97, 101, 114, 172
Public Policy, 113, 172
Pulmonary, 140, 146, 160, 172, 182
Pulmonary Artery, 140, 172, 182

Pulmonary hypertension, 146, 172
Pulse, 7, 23, 54, 163, 172

Q
Quality of Life, 8, 172

R
Race, 4, 150, 163, 172
Racemic, 150, 172
Radiation, 147, 151, 157, 172, 173, 183
Radio Waves, 149, 173
Radioactive, 156, 158, 165, 173
Radiopharmaceutical, 153, 173
Randomized, 22, 28, 34, 40, 56, 57, 70, 75, 87, 89, 150, 173
Receptivity, 9, 12, 17, 173
Receptor, 12, 14, 17, 19, 24, 38, 48, 72, 93, 95, 96, 138, 148, 150, 173, 176
Receptors, Steroid, 13, 173
Recombinant, 17, 20, 26, 40, 46, 75, 106, 173
Rectum, 138, 141, 144, 149, 153, 160, 172, 173
Recurrence, 47, 140, 173
Red Nucleus, 139, 173
Reductase, 43, 72, 173
Refer, 1, 145, 151, 161, 173, 175
Refraction, 173, 177
Regimen, 60, 75, 150, 173
Remission, 140, 173
Renin, 60, 64, 138, 173
Renin-Angiotensin System, 64, 173
Reproduction Techniques, 31, 64, 170, 173
Reproductive cells, 153, 173
Reproductive system, 8, 21, 24, 174
Resection, 12, 13, 47, 51, 54, 55, 93, 174
Respiration, 142, 163, 174
Retina, 146, 166, 174
Retinal, 32, 166, 174
Retinal Vein, 32, 174
Retinal Vein Occlusion, 32, 174
Retinoblastoma, 116, 174
Retinol, 174
Retroperitoneal, 136, 174
Retrospective, 36, 46, 55, 174
Retrospective study, 46, 55, 174
Rhodopsin, 166, 174
Ribonucleic acid, 39, 174
Risk factor, 4, 5, 7, 11, 97, 171, 174
Rod, 140, 144, 174
Rubber, 135, 175

S
Salivary, 149, 167, 175
Salivary glands, 149, 175

Saponins, 175, 177
Sclerosis, 116, 139, 175
Screening, 144, 175
Sebaceous, 175, 183
Sebaceous gland, 175, 183
Secretion, 6, 7, 10, 16, 21, 22, 23, 25, 32, 35, 37, 38, 39, 45, 57, 62, 71, 72, 80, 89, 92, 94, 147, 154, 156, 157, 158, 159, 161, 163, 164, 175, 183
Secretory, 12, 16, 21, 60, 175
Seizures, 13, 141, 167, 168, 175
Semen, 171, 175
Seminiferous tubule, 137, 158, 175
Semisynthetic, 152, 175
Senescence, 93, 175
Septal, 175
Septum, 17, 175
Septum Pellucidum, 175
Sequencing, 175, 179
Serine, 27, 175, 180
Serotonin, 165, 175
Serum, 7, 11, 15, 18, 21, 48, 56, 57, 60, 61, 65, 71, 74, 87, 88, 89, 93, 132, 145, 154, 161, 163, 176
Sex Characteristics, 136, 137, 172, 176, 179
Sex Determination, 117, 176
Sex Hormone-Binding Globulin, 49, 62, 64, 176
Shivering, 176, 179
Signal Transduction, 19, 72, 158, 176
Skeletal, 101, 137, 144, 164, 176
Skeleton, 159, 171, 176
Skull, 176, 179
Small intestine, 144, 156, 159, 176
Smooth muscle, 141, 146, 173, 176, 178
Social Environment, 172, 176
Sodium, 163, 176, 177, 182
Sodium Channels, 177, 182
Somatic, 136, 162, 163, 168, 177
Somatic cells, 162, 163, 177
Somatostatin, 59, 71, 73, 177
Sound wave, 149, 177
Specialist, 124, 149, 177
Species, 23, 25, 152, 153, 156, 162, 163, 172, 177, 178, 181, 183
Specificity, 136, 177
Spectrum, 4, 10, 92, 159, 173, 177
Sperm, 20, 50, 137, 143, 173, 175, 177
Spinal cord, 141, 143, 165, 168, 177
Spontaneous Abortion, 52, 170, 177
Sporadic, 174, 177
Steel, 144, 177

Sterilization, 12, 177
Steroid, 9, 11, 13, 17, 23, 24, 33, 40, 41, 70, 92, 101, 137, 147, 153, 173, 175, 177
Stillbirth, 170, 178
Stimulus, 150, 152, 178, 179
Stomach, 135, 149, 152, 153, 154, 156, 159, 164, 176, 178
Stool, 144, 160, 178
Stress, 93, 142, 147, 164, 175, 178
Stroke, 21, 90, 112, 142, 178
Stroma, 82, 93, 178
Stromal, 9, 66, 151, 178
Stromal Cells, 9, 178
Subclinical, 7, 88, 158, 175, 178
Subcutaneous, 48, 135, 150, 178
Subspecies, 177, 178
Substance P, 171, 175, 178
Substrate, 14, 93, 152, 178
Superovulation, 70, 81, 178
Supplementation, 71, 178
Suppression, 6, 10, 16, 30, 41, 61, 92, 137, 147, 178
Sympathomimetic, 150, 152, 165, 178
Symphysis, 143, 172, 178
Symptomatic, 13, 178
Synapse, 136, 170, 178, 181
Synapsis, 178, 179
Synaptic, 23, 165, 176, 178
Synchrony, 35, 179
Synergistic, 171, 179
Systemic, 17, 141, 152, 158, 179, 181
Systolic, 157, 179

T
Telangiectasia, 117, 179
Telencephalon, 140, 143, 179
Temporal, 13, 62, 179
Temporal Lobe, 13, 179
Teratoma, 53, 179
Testicle, 154, 179
Testis, 11, 137, 152, 179
Testosterone, 6, 10, 16, 18, 22, 24, 35, 39, 62, 64, 72, 80, 132, 137, 161, 173, 176, 179
Thalamic, 139, 179
Thalamic Diseases, 139, 179
Theca Cells, 8, 16, 23, 85, 161, 179
Thermogenesis, 59, 179
Third Ventricle, 157, 179
Threshold, 49, 71, 73, 157, 179
Thrombin, 153, 172, 179, 180
Thrombomodulin, 172, 180
Thrombophilia, 52, 180
Thrombosis, 172, 178, 180

Thromboxanes, 139, 180
Thyroid, 157, 180, 182
Thyrotropin, 157, 180
Tissue Plasminogen Activator, 29, 180
Tolerance, 135, 154, 180
Tomography, 145, 180
Tone, 38, 180
Tonus, 180
Toxaemia, 170, 180
Toxemia, 81, 180
Toxic, iv, 151, 180
Toxicology, 114, 180
Toxins, 138, 158, 180
Trace element, 143, 181
Traction, 144, 181
Transcription Factors, 24, 26, 181
Transduction, 176, 181
Transfection, 26, 140, 153, 181
Transgenes, 19, 181
Translational, 7, 181
Translocation, 16, 24, 181
Transmitter, 135, 150, 162, 165, 181
Transplantation, 144, 151, 161, 181
Treatment Outcome, 50, 181
Tricuspid Atresia, 146, 181
Triptorelin, 73, 181
Troglitazone, 21, 101, 181
Trophic, 14, 181
Trophoblast, 12, 140, 181
Tuberous Sclerosis, 117, 181
Tumor marker, 140, 181
Type 2 diabetes, 4, 5, 15, 22, 75, 101, 105, 181
Tyrosine, 150, 182

U

Ultrasonography, 45, 54, 57, 58, 182
Unconscious, 157, 182
Urethra, 167, 171, 182
Urinary, 34, 44, 51, 74, 75, 83, 169, 180, 182
Urinary Plasminogen Activator, 180, 182
Urine, 140, 149, 154, 155, 159, 169, 172, 182
Uterus, 135, 143, 147, 148, 151, 162, 167, 171, 174, 182

V

Vaccine, 135, 182
Vagina, 143, 162, 174, 182
Vaginal, 7, 68, 120, 182
Valproic Acid, 28, 74, 182
Vascular, 141, 158, 166, 169, 182
Vasodilation, 88, 182
Vasodilator, 150, 182
Vein, 137, 159, 165, 174, 182
Venous, 172, 181, 182
Ventricle, 139, 146, 172, 179, 181, 182
Ventricular, 146, 179, 181, 182
Vesicular, 153, 155, 182
Veterinary Medicine, 113, 183
Vinyl Chloride, 18, 183
Virilism, 15, 156, 183
Virilization, 58, 132, 183
Virus, 139, 169, 181, 183
Vitamin A, 158, 174, 183
Vitro, 9, 12, 15, 16, 19, 20, 21, 23, 43, 45, 55, 56, 61, 63, 65, 66, 71, 73, 74, 79, 81, 82, 93, 95, 142, 151, 153, 158, 181, 183
Vivo, 15, 16, 19, 21, 24, 46, 183

W

White blood cell, 138, 161, 163, 164, 183
Womb, 174, 182, 183

X

Xenograft, 138, 183
X-ray, 145, 146, 165, 183

Y

Yeasts, 168, 183

Z

Zona Pellucida, 20, 183
Zygote, 146, 183
Zymogen, 172, 183